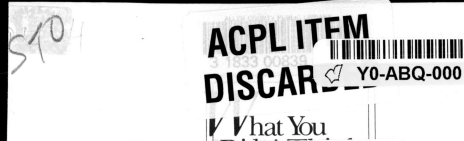

What You Didn't Think to Ask Your Obstetrician

All Your Questions Answered

Raymond I. Poliakin, M.D.

CONTEMPORARY
BOOKS, INC.
CHICAGO ▪ NEW YORK

Library of Congress Cataloging-in-Publication Data

Poliakin, Raymond.
   What you didn't think to ask your obstetrician.

   1. Pregnancy—Miscellanea.   2. Obstetrics—Popular
works.   I. Title.   [DNLM: 1. Obstetrics—popular works.
2. Pregnancy—popular works.   WQ 150 P766w]
RG556.P65   1987   618.2   87-19917
ISBN 0-8092-4721-6 (pbk.)

Published by Contemporary Books, Inc.
180 North Michigan Avenue, Chicago, Illinois 60601
Manufactured in the United States of America
Library of Congress Catalog Card Number: 87-19917
International Standard Book Number: 0-8092-4721-6

Published simultaneously in Canada by Beaverbooks, Ltd.
195 Allstate Parkway, Valleywood Business Park
Markham, Ontario L3R 4T8 Canada

2309153

To my mother and father
for their love, support, and devotion
throughout the years

Contents

1 Office Visits and Early Considerations   1
2 Growth and Development of the Fetus   7
3 Common Complaints During Pregnancy   13
4 Diet and Nutrition   28
5 Health and Fitness Concerns   37
6 Drugs and Medications   49
7 Special Tests   57
8 Obstetrical Complications of Pregnancy   70
9 Medical Complications of Pregnancy   91
10 Labor and Delivery   106
11 Cesarean Section   131
12 Postpartum   138
13 Pregnancy in Women Over 35   152
14 Myths   155
    Index   159

1 Office Visits and Early Considerations

Q *What happens at your first prenatal visit?*

A The doctor will take a complete history, including any or all of the following:
- Past medical history
- Past surgical history
- Gynecological history
- Obstetrical history
- Allergies
- Medications
- Family history
- Social history
- First day of your last menstrual period (LMP)

Your doctor will discuss any problems associated with your past history and basic problems and solutions that may arise during your pregnancy. Bring a list of questions that you may want answered. He will prescribe a prenatal vitamin and explain what will happen during your follow-up visits and your appointment schedule based on your LMP.

Your weight and blood pressure will be taken and recorded as a baseline. You may be asked to urinate before your pelvic exam, because the bladder sits on top of the uterus and a full

1

bladder makes for both an uncomfortable exam for you and a difficult and sometimes misleading exam for the doctor. A physical exam will be performed including a breast and pelvic exam. A pap smear, if due, will be performed. Blood will be taken for the following tests: CBC, VDRL, rubella, blood type, and Rh titer.

Q *Why is the pelvic exam performed?*

A The pelvic exam tells us many important facts. First, it confirms your pregnancy and the length of your pregnancy thus far. The doctor will also be able to discover any abnormalities of the uterus, such as fibroid tumors (a benign tumor of the muscles of the uterus), congenital abnormalities of the uterus, cysts or tumors of the ovary, or the presence of an ectopic pregnancy (see Chapter 8). The doctor will also measure the birth canal and estimate its adequacy for passage of your baby.

Q *What does the CBC (complete blood count) tell us?*

A It measures the number of red blood cells (RBC) in your body, along with hemoglobin, the oxygen-carrying protein found in the RBC, and the hematocrit (the percentage of RBCs relative to plasma—the fluid that allows the RBCs to flow in your vessels). If these are low, you are anemic and require treatment with iron. The number of white blood cells and platelets are also recorded.

Q *What is the VDRL?*

A This is a screening test for syphilis. Syphilis during pregnancy can cause a myriad of congenital anomalies in your fetus, but not if the disease is treated early in pregnancy.

Q *What is the Rubella test?*

A Rubella is German measles. This test tells us if you are immune to the virus that causes German measles. This virus can cause many abnormalities in your fetus. If you are immune to the virus, you do not have to worry if you are exposed to it. If you are not immune to rubella, this test serves two purposes: First, if you are exposed to German measles, another rubella test can be drawn to verify if you were actually infected. Second, a rubella vaccine will be given postpartum as an immunization for further pregnancies.

Q *Why are the blood type and Rh titer drawn?*

A The Rh titer is the most important part of this test during early pregnancy. The Rh antigen is a small protein found on the RBC. Rh positive means this protein is present. A woman with Rh negative blood will have further tests during the course of her pregnancy. This will be discussed later.

The incidence of Rh negative blood is as follows:
- Whites—13%
- Blacks—7% to 8%
- Asians—1%

Q *How often are the follow-up visits?*

A The schedule of visits is often as follows:
- Every 4 weeks until 20 weeks
- Every 3 weeks from 20 to 30 weeks
- Every 2 weeks from 30 to 36 weeks
- Weekly until delivery after 36 weeks

Q *What does the doctor do during the follow-up visits?*

A The doctor will always:
- Check your first morning urine
- Check your weight and blood pressure
- Measure the size of your uterus
- After 30 weeks, examine for the position of the fetus
- Listen for fetal heart tones
- Educate and answer questions
- Perform special screening tests

Q *Why is the first morning urine tested?*

A The doctor tests the first morning urine for the presence of sugar, protein, and nitrites. About one-sixth of pregnant women will have sugar in their urine normally; however, since this also occurs in diabetes mellitus, a test would then be performed for this disorder. If protein is found in your urine, you may have a problem with your kidneys. The nitrite test screens for a possible urinary tract infection.

Q *Why is the uterus measured?*

A The uterus is measured to ascertain proper growth of the fetus and to alert your doctor to any possible problems, such as miscarriage, blighted ovum, molar pregnancy, twins, or a growth-retarded fetus.

Q *How is the uterus measured?*

A Until the 12th week of pregnancy, the uterus is measured by pelvic examination. The uterus can first be felt abdominally at about 14 weeks. Between 14 and 20 weeks the uterus is measured in relation to the belly button. After 20 weeks a tape measure is used to measure the distance from the top of your pubic bone to the top of your uterus (the fundus). This length, measured in centimeters, correlates with the week of your pregnancy until the 32nd week.

Q *Do I have pelvic exams during each office visit?*

A Most physicians perform a pelvic exam during the initial office visit, and again at the end of your pregnancy. The pelvic exams at 38 weeks and beyond are used by your doctor to assess the ripeness of your cervix, an indication that your pregnancy is mature and ready for the birth of your baby!

Q *When can you first hear the fetal heart tones?*

A With a doptone, an instrument that uses ultrasonic waves, the fetal heart can be heard between 10 and 12 weeks. With the Delee-Hillis stethoscope the fetal heart can be heard at 20 weeks.

Q *What other screening tests might be performed?*

A Alphafetoprotein, amniocentesis, chorionic villus sampling, diabetes screening, ultrasound, in addition to another hematocrit and Rh titer (if you are Rh negative) may be performed later in your pregnancy.

CHILDBIRTH CLASSES

Q *Should I take a prepared childbirth class?*

A If this is your first pregnancy, yes! There are many benefits to attending a prepared childbirth class. Foremost is the psychological preparation for the pain of labor. If you are aware of what to expect and ready yourself, you will deal with the pain of uterine contractions much more effectively. Women who take a prepared childbirth class require less pain medication, less often, during labor. Of course you do not have to take these classes just to avoid the administration of medications during labor. You may take these classes with the thought of having an epidural throughout labor. These classes also review the anatomy of the female reproductive system, physiology and mechanics of labor, nutrition during pregnancy and postpartum, breast-feeding, cesarean sections, fetal monitoring, and hospital procedures. There are two schools of prepared childbirth—Lamaze and Bradley.

Q *What is the Lamaze method?*

A The Lamaze method, or the Psychoprophylactic Method (PPM), relies on the principle of conditioning against pain. By practicing relaxation techniques, the woman will be able to concentrate on relieving tension when a labor contraction (pain) occurs. This is done, with the help of her partner, by utilizing different breathing patterns during labor. It is often a rewarding team effort, in which couples successfully work together through each contraction.

Q *What is the Bradley method?*

A The Bradley method is a stricter form of childbirth class, which emphasizes a "natural" birth with the avoidance of any medication for pain. This method teaches women to concentrate on the pain instead of avoiding it by using breathing patterns. Several methods of relaxation are taught and women are encouraged to use the method which best suits them. The partner acts as a support person who encourages the woman during labor with positive statements. This method also recommends that the couple create their own unique birth plan for labor and delivery and discuss it with their doctor.

Q *How are the classes offered?*

A The classes are offered once a week for 6 to 8 weeks. Each class is about 3 hours long.

Q *When do I take these classes?*

A Plan on taking the class at about your 30th week, so that you can finish the classes before you deliver. Also, you will have plenty of time to practice what you have learned in class.

WARNING SIGNS

Q *Are there warning signs that I should be aware of and notify my doctor about?*

A There are several complications of pregnancy that may occur. Fortunately, most pregnancies progress without difficulty. However, if you experience any of these symptoms, call your doctor immediately:
- Vaginal spotting not related to intercourse
- Vaginal bleeding
- A gush of fluid or a steady flow of fluid from your vagina
- Continuous vomiting
- Frequent and painful urination
- Fever (over 100.4°F) and chills with flank pain or abdominal pain not accompanied by diarrhea or the flu
- Labor contractions occurring at least 10 minutes apart before your 37th week of pregnancy
- Severe persistent headache
- Blurred vision
- Sudden swelling in your hands and face
- Sudden and rapid weight gain
- Decreased urination despite normal or increased drinking habits
- Right upper abdominal pain
- Decreased or absent fetal movement for 24 hours in the third trimester

2 Growth and Development of the Fetus

Q *How long does the average pregnancy last?*

A The average pregnancy or gestation lasts 280 days or 40 weeks or 10 lunar (4-week) months or 9 calendar months. Obstetricians calculate the pregnancy from the first day of your last menstrual period (LMP). Ovulation and conception, however, do not occur until 14 days later, so the fetus grows for about 266 days. Your pregnancy is also divided into 3 equal trimesters. The duration of each trimester is 13 weeks or 3 calendar months.

Q *How do you calculate the delivery date?*

A You may calculate the delivery date by using Nagele's rule: subtract 3 months from your LMP and add 7 days. For example, if your LMP was December 22, your due date would be September 29. The EDC (estimated date of confinement) is your due date. Your doctor will have a pregnancy wheel or a calculator to calculate your EDC. Calculation of the due date is based on a 28-day menstrual cycle with ovulation occurring on the 14th day. If your menstrual cycle is longer or shorter than 28 days, you must add (if longer) or subtract (if shorter) the corresponding number of days.

Q What are the chances of delivering on the EDC?

A About 5% of women will have their delivery on the EDC. About 50% will deliver within one week and 80% will deliver within two weeks before or after the EDC.

Q Is the duration of the first pregnancy usually longer than subsequent pregnancies?

A No. Actually, women who have previously delivered tend to have slightly longer pregnancies.

Q If I previously delivered early or late, will I do so again?

A You have a good chance of doing so. Women tend to repeat their past history of delivery timing.

Q When does the fetus first move?

A It has been shown, using ultrasound, that the fetus twitches between 7 and 10 weeks, moves arms and legs at 10 to 12 weeks, and moves limbs, head, and torso by 16 weeks.

Q When will I first feel my baby move?

A Usually between the 16th and 20th weeks you may notice a slight fluttering in your abdomen that will become increasingly stronger as the days go by. The first feeling of fetal activity is called "quickening" and is your first perception that your fetus is alive.

Q What is the placenta?

A The placenta is an organ of the fetus, which serves many functions. It attaches to your uterus and is bathed by your blood, taking oxygen and nutrients to the fetus and returning fetal waste products back into your circulation for disposal. The placenta can also actively transport certain substances from your blood to the fetus, such as proteins and calcium, which are needed in greater amounts for growth. Most anything that gets into your circulation can get into the fetal bloodstream, including medication and drugs, if the molecules are small enough. Viruses can also pass through the placenta, but the placenta actively transports your antibodies to the fetus to provide immunity against disease. The placenta also produces several different hormones which are used to maintain and increase the growth of the fetus. One of these hormones is called human chorionic gonadotropin; this is the hormone measured in pregnancy tests.

Q *What is the umbilical cord?*

A The umbilical cord is the lifeline for your fetus. The umbilical cord attaches from the placenta to the umbilicus (navel or belly button) of the fetus. The umbilical cord contains three vessels—two arteries, and one vein. The umbilical vein carries oxygenated and nutrient-rich blood from the placenta to the fetus, and the umbilical arteries carry away oxygen-poor blood back to the placenta. These vessels are cushioned by a substance called Wharton's jelly and are all wrapped by amniotic membrane.

Q *What is the chorioamniotic sac?*

A The chorioamniotic sac is also known as the "amniotic sac" or "bag" or "membrane." This is the membrane that covers the inside of the placenta and uterus and surrounds the fetus and amniotic fluid.

Q *What is amniotic fluid?*

A This is the fluid that surrounds the fetus. At term there is about a quart of amniotic fluid present. Amniotic fluid is made from the fluid oozing across the membranes initially. In the second and third trimesters, amniotic fluid also comes from fetal urine. The fetus at term drinks about a pint of amniotic fluid a day, about as much milk as a newborn drinks. The fetus must also urinate that much to keep the amount of amniotic fluid present in balance. There is also a constant transfer of fluid back and forth through the membranes equaling about 8 ounces an hour.

Q *What happens during the first month of pregnancy?*

A Remember that you do not become pregnant until after

ovulation, which takes place on about day 14 of a 28-day menstrual cycle. Fertilization of your egg by your partner's sperm follows on that day. During the next 6 days the fertilized egg, or zygote, travels down your fallopian tube and divides into 16 cells (morula) by day 17 and to the many-celled blastocyst by day 20. The blastocyst attaches to your uterus on day 20 or 21 of your cycle, or 6 to 7 days after ovulation. This is called implantation. On the 22nd day the blastocyst separates into what will become the placenta and your baby, called the trophoblast and embryo, respectively. On day 26, the circulation between your uterus and the placenta has been established and the amniotic cavity has formed. On day 28, the 14-day-old embryo is composed of three different cell layers and has formed the chorioamniotic sac. The pregnancy is now completely surrounded by specialized uterine tissue called decidua. The embryo is about 2 millimeters, or $\frac{1}{12}$ of an inch, long.

Q How big is my baby at 6 weeks' gestation (6 weeks after the first day of your last menstrual period)?

A The embryo is $\frac{1}{6}$ of an inch long and weighs $\frac{1}{70}$ of an ounce. The embryo's chin rests on its chest and limb buds have formed. There is a prominent tail. The heart has started beating by the fifth week, and by the end of 6 weeks has four chambers. The beginning of the brain and spinal cord has formed. In fact, all major organs have begun to form. The embryo is now floating in amniotic fluid and may be seen by ultrasound.

Q How big is my baby at 8 weeks?

A Your fetus is about one inch long and weighs $\frac{1}{30}$ of an ounce. The fetus is about one-half head and you can see its eyes, ears, nose, and mouth. The intestines are in the umbilical cord. The fingers and toes have formed and the tail has almost disappeared. Your uterus is about the size of an orange.

Q How big is my baby at 12 weeks?

A Your fetus is $3\frac{1}{2}$ inches long and weighs about $\frac{1}{2}$ ounce. The fingers have started growing nails. The arms and legs can now bend and have reached their relative length in comparison to the rest of the body. The intestines are now back in the abdomen. The face has become more human looking. There are about 1½ ounces of amniotic fluid. Your uterus is about the size of a cantaloupe.

Q *How big is my baby at 16 weeks?*

A Your fetus is 6 inches long and weighs 4 ounces. You can now see a rudimentary penis or vagina. Scalp hair has begun to form and your fetus is actively moving about. It has breathing movements and has begun to swallow amniotic fluid. The fetus also starts urinating now. Bones have started to form. The top of your uterus, called the fundus, can be felt midway between your pubic bone and belly button. There are about 8 ounces of amniotic fluid. Thumb-sucking can begin now.

Q *How big is my baby at 20 weeks?*

A Your fetus is almost 10 inches long and weighs about 12 ounces. The head comprises one-third of its length. Vernix caseosa, a white cheesy material composed of oil and old fetal skin cells, covers the fetus protecting its skin from becoming macerated by the amniotic fluid. The toenails begin to develop. The face is fully developed now. There are about 13 ounces of amniotic fluid.

Q *How big is my baby at 24 weeks?*

A Your fetus is 12 inches long and weighs 1¼ pounds. The skin is wrinkled and has very delicate hair called lanugo growing all over its body. Eyebrows and eyelashes appear now, too. Fat starts developing. Breathing movements start, but the lungs are not well developed. Survival if born now is rare.

Q *How big is my baby at 28 weeks?*

A Your fetus is 14 inches long and weighs about 2¼ pounds. The skin is now red and shiny and has lost its wrinkles due to the deposition of more fat. The body is still lean and trim though. The eyelids have opened now. Your fetus may appear to move less but it doesn't; there is just less room for it to move around. Survival if born now is much better.

Q *How big is my baby at 32 weeks?*

A Your fetus is about 16 inches long and weighs 3¾ pounds. If the baby is born prematurely now, his or her chance of surviving is over 80%.

Q *How big is my baby at 36 weeks?*

A Your fetus is 18 inches long and weighs 5½ pounds. The body is now plump and the lanugo hairs have begun to disappear. The fingernails and toenails reach to the tips. The skin is pink and smooth. If a male, the testes have begun to descend into the scrotum.

Q *How big is my baby at 40 weeks?*

A The average length is 19½ inches and your baby may weigh from 6 to 10 pounds or more. The average weight is 7½ pounds.

Q *How big is the placenta at term?*

A The placenta, also known as the afterbirth, weighs about 1½ pounds. It is flat and circular in shape, with a diameter of 7½ inches, and is about 1 inch thick. The size and weight of the placenta are proportional to the size and weight of the baby.

Q *How long is the umbilical cord at term?*

A Though the length varies, the average length of the umbilical cord is 21 inches. The more active the fetus, the longer the cord. The cord's diameter is about 1 inch.

3 Common Complaints During Pregnancy

Q *Why do I urinate so frequently at the beginning of my pregnancy?*

A First, we must understand the anatomy of the bladder and its relationship to the uterus. The bladder rests on top of the uterus. In the first trimester, as the uterus grows, the bladder is stretched. A woman's brain perceives this signal as the sensation of a full bladder. In addition, the rate of urine production is increased.

Q *Why am I urinating frequently at the end of my pregnancy?*

A You may notice there is a decrease in the frequency of urination in the middle of your pregnancy, and then an increase again after 32 weeks, due to the increased pressure of the bladder by the growing head of the fetus.

Q *Is it common to leak urine when I cough, laugh, sneeze, jump, or run during pregnancy?*

A Yes, this is very common and is due to the changing position of the bladder throughout pregnancy. Kegel exercises (explained below) may decrease the frequency of this sometimes embarrassing condition. Usually this annoyance disappears a few months postpartum.

Q *What are Kegel exercises?*

A Kegel exercises are designed to strengthen the muscles of your pelvic floor to gain better control of your bladder both during pregnancy and postpartum. To do these exercises, contract and loosen the muscles around your vagina, much like you would if you were starting and stopping the flow of urine during urination (you may practice this while urinating too). Do sets of 10 or 20 each day—in the car at a red light or during a commercial break while watching TV.

Q *In early pregnancy is mild uterine cramping normal?*

A Yes, it is. This cramping is called *Braxton-Hicks* contractions and can be mildly uncomfortable. This cramping can begin as early as 8 weeks. If the cramps are severe or accompanied by vaginal bleeding, contact your obstetrician.

Q *In early pregnancy, is it normal to have pains going down to the groin?*

A Yes. This is called the *round ligament syndrome.* These ligaments stretch as the uterus grows, and this stretching is perceived as pain.

Q *In mid- to late pregnancy, is it common to have pain down the back of my leg(s)?*

A Yes. This is due to the increased pressure of the weight of your pregnant uterus on the sciatic nerve which supplies this area. You may also experience hip pain, due to the combination of the weight of your pregnant uterus and your weight gain.

Q *Why are my breasts tender?*

A The increase in the production of estrogen causes the breast tissue to swell and become tender. This tenderness is usually most annoying during the first 6 to 12 weeks of your pregnancy.

Q *When will my breasts begin to grow?*

A Beginning at 6 weeks your breasts will begin to enlarge due to water retention in the breast tissue. After 8 weeks, the milk glands and ducts begin to enlarge along with the increased growth of fatty tissue.

Q *What other changes will occur in my breasts?*

A Due to the increase in tissue in the breast, there will be an increase in the blood supply. You may note the appearance of bluish veins in the skin on your breasts. Your areola and nipples will darken. The nipples will become much larger and erectile to accommodate feeding your baby. If there is a great increase in the size of your breasts, you may develop stretch marks.

Q *How big will my breasts grow?*

A Every woman is different, but expect at least a two-cup change and a ½-pound increase in the weight of each breast.

Q *What is colostrum?*

A Colostrum is a thick, yellowish fluid discharged from the breast. Colostrum may appear anytime after the first trimester, with its quantity increasing after delivery. Colostrum nourishes the baby before your milk comes in. It also contains antibodies that will provide your baby with immunity to diseases to which you have resistance.

Q *What should I do to prevent or treat caked nipples?*

A Caked nipples are caused by colostrum that has dried on your nipples. If you are leaking colostrum, place a cotton or gauze pad into your bra to absorb the fluid. If your nipples are already caked with dried colostrum, wash your breasts with warm water only, two or three times a day.

Q *What causes lower back pains?*

A As your pregnancy progresses, the size and weight of the uterus changes your center of balance. To compensate for this change, your posture changes—you lean backward, making the lower muscles in your back work harder, causing muscle strain.

Q *When will it occur, if ever?*

A Usually anytime after 20 weeks.

Q *What can you do to relieve this backache?*

A For prevention and relief:
- Sleep on a firm mattress.
- Sit on a straight-back chair and try not to slouch on a couch.
- Maintain an erect posture.
- When bending down, bend from the knees, not from the waist.
- Wear comfortable shoes (the shoes don't have to be flat, but spike heels may aggravate the pain).
- Improve your posture by standing next to a wall, making sure your head and shoulders, back and buttocks are touching the wall at the same time for 5 to 10 seconds 5 to 10 times a day.
- Do pelvic rock exercises.
- You may use a heating pad for 10 minutes at a time.
- A maternity girdle may be useful, especially if you have poor abdominal muscle tone.
- If your backache is severe, you may need more extensive care by your doctor.

Q *Is constipation common during pregnancy?*

A Yes, it is. It occurs in about 30% of pregnant women.

Q *When will constipation most commonly occur?*

A During the first and third trimesters.

Q *What causes constipation during pregnancy?*

A Decreased intestinal motion and/or increased absorption of water by the intestine, due to the increased amount of hormone (in this case progesterone), will cause constipation and harder stools. Iron found in your prenatal vitamins may cause constipation. Your enlarging uterus may press down on your large intestine and cause a slowdown.

Q What can I do to prevent or relieve constipation?

A
- Drink at least 8 glasses of fluids a day.
- Eat vegetables, fruits, and bran.
- Increase your physical activity.
- Ask your doctor if you could use a laxative such as Milk of Magnesia, Senekot, or Dialose Plus.
- Avoid foods such as bananas, rice, apples, or toast (this is the BRAT diet used if you have diarrhea!).

Q When do leg cramps occur during a pregnancy?

A Leg cramps occur after the first trimester, becoming more common until the last month of pregnancy when they occur infrequently.

Q When are they most likely to occur?

A At night when you are sleeping or lying down.

Q What causes leg cramps?

A Either too little calcium or too much phosphorus in your diet can cause leg cramps. Calcium is found in milk and cheese, so is phosphorus. Phosphorus is also found in red meat. Or, you may be absorbing calcium poorly. Inactivity and poor circulation, caused by the pressure of your growing uterus on the great vessels, are contributing factors.

Q What can I do to prevent leg cramps?

A
- Drink no more than one pint of milk a day.
- Limit the amount of red meat in your diet to one serving a day.
- Supplement your diet with 500 to 1,000 milligrams of calcium in the form of calcium lactate or carbonate.
- Shake your legs for 30 seconds each night before going to sleep.
- Raise the foot of your bed 6 inches.
- Sleep on your side, not on your back.

Q What can I do when I get a leg cramp?

A
- Turn over on your side or stand up to increase circulation to your legs.

- Point your foot towards your face to stretch the calf muscle.
- Rub and/or apply heat to your calf.

Q *Why did I become dizzy when I got out of bed this morning?*

A During pregnancy you may notice that your blood pressure is lower due to hormonal changes that cause your blood vessels to dilate. The vessels do not constrict as quickly or as efficiently in response to a change in your position. Therefore, standing up too fast does not allow your circulatory system to adjust in time, not enough blood and oxygen reach your brain, and you will feel faint. In addition, you may be anemic, so the oxygen-carrying capacity of your blood will be reduced, and, after an overnight fast, low blood sugar may also compound this problem.

Q *What can I do to prevent this dizziness?*

A Inform your doctor, who may want to test you for anemia and prescribe iron therapy. When getting out of bed, sit up and wait 15 seconds, then hang your legs off the bed and wait 15 seconds, stand and wait 15 seconds, and then start walking. If you notice that dizziness during the day is relieved by a snack, drink a glass of orange juice before getting out of bed.

Q *Why do I become dizzy if I stand in one place for too long?*

A Standing in place and not moving allows your blood to pool in your legs. To avoid this, walk in place; your calf muscles will help pump your blood back to your heart.

Q *Is it normal to be tired all the time?*

A Yes, it may begin in the first trimester and linger throughout your pregnancy.

Q *What causes this fatigue?*

A The increased level of progesterone produces a sedative effect. Fatigue is also one of the characteristic signs of anemia.

Q *What should I do?*

A Tell your doctor. He will test for anemia. If you are anemic, iron therapy will be prescribed. You will feel better in about 5 weeks. If you are not anemic, you need more rest; go to sleep earlier and, if you can, take a nap or lie down during the day.

Q *Is flatulence (gas) more common during pregnancy?*

A Yes. Both flatulence and belching can increase during pregnancy. Intestinal gas will cause your abdomen to distend and you may feel bloated. To minimize these feelings, avoid foods such as cabbage and beans.

Q *Does pregnancy cause my gums to bleed and swell?*

A Yes. This is called pregnancy gingivitis and occurs in at least 30% of pregnant mothers. It can begin as early as the first month of pregnancy and can become progressively worse. Your gums will return to their normal state 1 to 2 months after delivery, however.

Q *What causes pregnancy gingivitis?*

A A combination of an increase in progesterone and inadequate oral hygiene.

Q *Can pregnancy gingivitis be prevented?*

A Not always, but the severity can be decreased with the use of a toothbrush and dental floss. Begin good oral hygiene early. If the inflammation and swelling are severe, permanent damage to your gums might occur.

Q *Can I grow hair in abnormal places during my pregnancy?*

A Yes. Many women will notice the increased growth of fine hairs on their face, arms, and legs. Occasionally, new pubic hair will grow in the midline of your lower abdomen up towards your navel.

Q *Will these hairs disappear?*

A Yes. Usually in 2 to 6 months following delivery, these hairs will disappear, but they can return with each new pregnancy.

Q *Do pregnant women commonly develop headaches?*

A Yes, and they may occur throughout your pregnancy. The possible causes are numerous—emotional tension, sinusitis, eyestrain, fatigue, and anemia.

Q *How are headaches treated during pregnancy?*

A Conservative therapy is always the initial step. Try lying down in a dark room and relax. A cold or hot compress may aid in relief. Acetaminophen (Tylenol) or aspirin may be used during pregnancy, but ask your doctor first before self-prescribing medications.

Q *Sometimes I feel my heart pounding. How come?*

A This is a common disturbance during the last trimester. It is due to the increased blood volume and increased work performed by your heart. If the problem becomes frequent, tell your doctor. When it occurs, sit or lie down and relax; the episode usually lasts only a few seconds.

Q *How common is heartburn during pregnancy?*

A It affects up to 75% of pregnant women, usually beginning in the second trimester and becoming more frequent thereafter. About 25% of these women will experience it every day.

Q *What causes heartburn during pregnancy?*

A The increase in progesterone causes the stomach to empty into the intestines at a slower rate, allowing acid to enter the esophagus—the tube that connects the mouth to the stomach. As the pregnant uterus grows, it pushes into the stomach giving it less space and increasing the frequency of your symptoms.

Q *How can I decrease the frequency of heartburn?*

A • Eat several small meals during the day.

- After meals, sit or walk; don't lie down.
- Sleep on your side or if you sleep on your back, prop up your head and back with several pillows.

Q *What can I use to treat heartburn?*

A Antacids are the treatment of choice during pregnancy. Avoid preparations that contain sodium which can lead to uncomfortable water retention. Antacids may be taken one hour before and two hours after meals and at bedtime.

Q *Why do pregnant women develop hemorrhoids (piles)?*

A Hemorrhoids are distended vessels or varicose veins located in the anus. They are caused by a combination of the increased blood volume and growing weight of the pregnant uterus on the great vessels. Hemorrhoids appear to be hereditary. They usually appear in the third trimester or during the second stage of labor, as a consequence of your pushing efforts.

Q *Are hemorrhoids dangerous?*

A No, just uncomfortable and annoying. Hemorrhoids make their appearance known by causing rectal pain, itching, swelling, and/or bleeding. The bleeding can range from spotting to a large amount, which is self-limiting. If you are unsure of the source of your bleeding, rectal or vaginal, contact your doctor.

Q *How can I prevent hemorrhoids?*

A
- Avoid constipation.
- Avoid hard stools.
- Practice your Kegel exercises.

Q *What can I do to treat the hemorrhoids?*

A Replace all hemorrhoids protruding out of your anus with gentle finger pressure as soon as you discover one. Hot sitz baths two or three times a day may be soothing. Preparation H may be used during pregnancy; it does not contain a topical anesthetic agent.

Q *How common are nausea and vomiting (morning sickness) in the first trimester of pregnancy?*

A About 50% of pregnant women experience some degree of nausea. Morning sickness first appears at about 6 to 8 weeks into your pregnancy and may last until 12 weeks.

Q *What can I do to relieve my feelings of nausea?*

A Nausea occurs most commonly on an empty stomach. Since you are not eating while you sleep, nausea is most common in the morning—hence the name morning sickness. To prevent nausea, try to eat small, frequent meals throughout the day. Try to eat your meals slowly. Before you go to sleep at night, eat a slice of turkey, chicken, or cheese. These high-protein foods are digested more slowly, keeping food in your stomach for a longer period of time. In the morning before you get out of bed, eat two or three crackers with some milk and then remain in bed for another 10 to 15 minutes. Also, you may want to avoid certain foods that are greasy and spicy. Nausea may be caused by your body reacting to the hormones of pregnancy, too little glycogen—a sugar stored in your liver— and not enough vitamin B_6. Try taking vitamin B_6 as follows: 200 milligrams at bedtime and 100 milligrams in the morning.

Q *I have tried all these suggestions, but I still vomit a few times a day. What can I do?*

A There are several medications that your doctor can prescribe, which may help. They are usually in suppository form. In addition to curtailing your nausea, they may also make you very sleepy.

Q *Is morning sickness harmful to me or my baby?*

A Nausea and occasional vomiting in early pregnancy is most annoying, but not harmful. In fact, recent studies have shown that women who experience morning sickness have *fewer* miscarriages and stillborns!

A very small minority of pregnant women may develop hyperemesis gravidarum or severe continuous vomiting in early pregnancy. This may lead to severe dehydration and is treated by hospitalization with an I.V. to replenish fluids and antinausea medications.

Q *I've had a stuffy nose ever since I became pregnant. Did I develop an allergy to myself?*

A Nasal stuffiness and nosebleeds are common and are due to swollen mucous membranes in the nasal passages. The swelling is caused by the increase in your blood circulation. You may also develop a chronic cough from a postnasal drip.

Q *How can I treat these symptoms?*

A Using a humidifier may reduce the frequency and severity of these problems. A nasal decongestant may be used under your doctor's direction.

Q *Are nosebleeds more common during pregnancy?*

A Yes. This is due to the increased number of new blood vessels in the mucous membranes of your nose and the increased circulation. The bleeding is almost always self-limiting. When a nosebleed does occur, apply a cold compress to your nose. A humidifier may help prevent nosebleeds.

Q *My fingernails keep breaking. Is this common?*

A Changes in your nails may occur as early as the sixth week of your pregnancy. Brittle nails due to thinning and softening of your nail and accelerated growth are common.

Q *What can I do to prevent this?*

A A diet with adequate amounts of protein and calcium will help keep your nails hard. Keep your nails short if they continue to break.

Q *Why do my hands feel numb and why do my fingers tingle?*

A Stretching the nerves in your neck that supply your hands causes this condition, which affects 5% to 10% of pregnant women. It is due to drooping your shoulders and affects both hands. Numbness is most common upon wakening in the morning and may persist after delivery by the constant carrying of your baby.

Q *How can I prevent this?*

A Practice good posture (see backaches earlier in this chapter).

Q *Why do the lateral three fingers of my hand burn and have a pins-and-needles sensation?*

A This is called the *carpal tunnel syndrome* and usually affects only one hand. It is caused by compression of the median nerve by the swelling of tissues in the wrist. This condition is more common near the end of pregnancy and usually disappears postpartum.

Q *What is the treatment for carpal tunnel syndrome?*

A
• Restrict your intake of salty foods.
• Raise your hands above your head when lying down.
• A wrist splint, called a neutral splint, can be prescribed by your doctor.

Q *Is it common to have shortness of breath or to hyperventilate?*

A A feeling of "air hunger" or shortness of breath can occur anytime during pregnancy. The cause is twofold. In the first two trimesters, the added supply of progesterone increases the sensitivity of the respiratory center in the brain to carbon dioxide, causing a faster breathing rate. In the third trimester, your growing uterus presses into your lungs and crowds them.

Q *How can I stop this feeling?*

A
• Raise your arms over your head.
• Sleep with several pillows under your head and back.
• Take long deep breaths and relax—remember, this is a normal change during pregnancy.

Q *What is the "mask of pregnancy"?*

A This condition (melasma, cholasma), which occurs in at least 70% of pregnant women, is a darkening of the skin over the upper lip, cheeks, nose, and/or forehead. The pattern is blotchy and caused by increased pigment deposits. It may appear anytime after the first trimester and usually disappears a few months after delivery. The sun will cause an even deeper color change, so use a sunscreen.

Q *What other skin changes are common during pregnancy?*

A There is also darkening of the areolas and nipples and a dark pigmented line extending from your pubic bone to your navel called the *linea nigra*. It appears at the end of the first trimester. You may also notice the appearance of small freckles and moles. "Spiders," small red capillaries, may appear most commonly on your chest. These blanch and fill when pressed and are due to the higher levels of estrogen. The appearance or disappearance of acne may be seen.

Q *Will these skin changes persist postpartum?*

A Fortunately, no. If melasma persists, try using bleaching creams with hydroquinone with or without retanoic acid.

Q *Will I get stretch marks?*

A My answer to this is always yes and I am correct 90% of the time. Stretch marks will occur to some degree most commonly on the abdomen, thighs, and breasts. These *striae* are caused by a breakup in the crosslinks of the tissue under the skin. Initially, they appear purple or reddish-pink, but their color fades to a silver and then white.

Q *What can I do to prevent stretch marks?*

A Nothing. Creams and oils will make your skin nice and soft but they will do nothing to prevent stretch marks.

Q *Is it normal for my skin to be itchy during pregnancy?*

A Yes, itching may occur to some degree in about 20% of pregnant women. A skin rash does not necessarily have to be present. The itching may occur over your entire body or be localized in one area, such as your abdomen. Itching is most intense at night, and during hot, humid times of the year.

Q What can be done to relieve the itching?

A
- Take baths with oatmeal soap and oil.
- Use an antipruritic lotion containing menthol.
- Topical steroids and antihistamines may be prescribed by your doctor.

Q Why am I producing so much saliva?

A There is an increased production of saliva by the salivary glands during pregnancy which may infrequently be excessive. This annoying condition may cause nausea, may persist throughout pregnancy, and then disappear postpartum. If too bothersome, ask your doctor about medicines used to treat this disorder.

Q Why are my ankles and feet swollen?

A This swelling is called edema and is actually excess water in these tissues. It occurs most commonly in the third trimester, due to the weight of the uterus pressing on the main veins. This pressure slows down the return of blood from your legs and allows the water in the vessels to move out into the surrounding tissue in your legs, most notably in your ankles and feet. Swelling is most common during hot weather.

Q How can I prevent or relieve this swelling?

A
- Try not to stand in place for long periods at a time. Move your feet and calves around; this helps pump the blood out of your legs.
- Restrict your intake of salty foods.
- Don't wear tight half-length nylons.
- If you are able to, keep your toes above your nose when sitting or lying down.

Q I have a vaginal discharge. Is it an infection?

A If the discharge burns, itches, has a bad odor, or makes your vulva red and swollen, you may have an infection. If you have none of these complaints, you have the normal increased vaginal secretions that occur during pregnancy. This discharge may be clear or white and becomes mucoid near term.

Q *When could I develop varicose veins?*

A Varicose veins occur commonly near the end of the second trimester. They are due to the pressure of the pregnant uterus on the main veins, slowing down the blood flow and distending the veins in the legs and/or vulva. The veins are easily distended, because their tone is already decreased by the effects of progesterone. Varicose veins tend to occur in families; ask your mother if she has them.

Q *What is the treatment for varicose veins during pregnancy?*

A Treatment during pregnancy is for the symptomatic relief of pain only, and usually includes the following:
- Try maternity support hose first. If this does not relieve your symptoms, you may be fitted with elastic stockings by your doctor.
- A pregnancy girdle will relieve tension in vulvar varicosities.
- When possible, keep your toes above your nose.
- Don't stand in one place for long periods at a time.

4 Diet and Nutrition

Q *Why do I have to gain weight during my pregnancy?*

A Pregnancy causes certain organs of the body to grow to support the developing fetus. Remember your baby also adds weight to your body. Studies have shown that the best outcome of a pregnancy—a healthy baby—occurs when the mother gains an adequate amount of weight. The weight is distributed as follows:

Baby	7½ pounds
Placenta	1½ pounds
Amniotic fluid	2 pounds
Uterus	2 pounds
Breasts	2 pounds
Blood	3½ pounds
Fluid	3 pounds
Fat	3 pounds
TOTAL	24½ pounds

Q *My prepregnancy weight was in the normal range. How much weight should I gain?*

A You should gain at least 24 pounds and no more than 35 pounds. This is easily achieved by a diet supplying 2,400 calories per day.

Q *I was underweight before I became pregnant. How much weight should I gain?*

A Underweight women should gain at least 30 pounds. These women tend to have smaller babies. Your increased weight gain will have a greater influence on the weight gain of your baby, bringing his or her weight into the normal range.

Q *I was very overweight before I became pregnant. How much weight should I gain?*

A There is no minimal weight gain for the overweight pregnant woman. However, you should be concerned with the quality of your diet. For you, proper nutrition and exercise as supervised by your doctor will assure good growth for your baby. Studies have shown that weight gain had little effect on the growth of these babies. But inadequate nutrition *will* have an effect on the development of your baby, so don't diet.

Q *What is the average weight gain during pregnancy?*

A For all prepregnancy weights, the average weight gain has been recorded at about 33 pounds in some studies. Don't be overly concerned with weight gain; you will gain weight. Place your emphasis on eating the proper foods.

Q *How many extra calories do I need daily during my pregnancy?*

A The Food and Nutrition Board has recommended an extra 300 calories per day. To maintain her weight before becoming pregnant, the average woman requires 2,000 calories per day. The 300 additional calories are an average throughout your pregnancy. Don't be worried if you are nauseous in the beginning of your pregnancy and can't eat. The need for additional calories is greater in the last trimester when you may consume a total caloric intake of 2,500 or more calories per day.

Q *How should my weight gain be distributed throughout my pregnancy?*

A
- First trimester—5 pounds
- Second trimester—10 pounds
- Third trimester—10 pounds

Q *How can I gain the weight?*

A Weight gain during pregnancy is easy. Putting the weight on properly is the hard part; a fast-food diet is not the way. Now that you are pregnant, it is time to prepare for parenthood by nourishing your baby properly. A well-rounded diet from the four basic food groups is the key to proper nutrition, caloric intake, and weight gain during pregnancy. If you eat the proper foods, according to your appetite, you will achieve these goals.

Q *Why should I eat a well-balanced diet?*

A A well-balanced diet will supply your body and growing fetus with the energy, proteins, vitamins, and minerals needed for proper development. The fetus will not be able to obtain all the essential nutrients from those already stored in your body, as was once believed to be true. Poor nutrition also increases the risk of complications during pregnancy, such as preterm labor and toxemia.

Q *What are the four basic food groups?*

A Milk, meat, fruits and vegetables, and grains. The following table illustrates the recommended daily servings before and during pregnancy:

Food Group	Before Pregnancy	During Pregnancy
Meat	2 servings	3 servings
Milk	2 servings	4 servings
Fruits and vegetables		
Vit. C source	daily	daily
Vit. A source	3–4/week	daily
Other	2–3 servings	2 servings
Grains	4 servings	4 servings

Q How much is one serving from the meat group?

A One serving is equivalent to:
    2–3 ounces of red meat, fish, or poultry
    2 eggs
    2 ounces of cheese
    1 cup canned or dried beans or peas
    1 cup of tofu
    ½ cup of nuts
    ¼ cup of peanut butter
    1 cup of garbanzo, lima, or kidney beans or lentils

Q Why should I eat foods from the meat group?

A Foods from the meat group supply you and your baby with protein, B vitamins, and iron. These nutrients are used to build and maintain bone, muscle, blood cells, skin, and nerves.

Q How much is one serving from the milk group?

A One serving is equivalent to:
    1 cup of milk—whole, skim, or nonfat
    1 cup of yogurt
    1 ounce of cheese
    1 cup of pudding
    2 cups of cottage cheese
    1 cup of ice milk
    1 milkshake
    1½ cups of ice cream

Q Why should I eat foods from the milk group?

A Foods from the milk group supply you and your baby with calcium, protein, vitamins A and D, and riboflavin. These nutrients are essential for strong bones and teeth, healthy skin, and good vision.

Q How much is one serving from the fruit and vegetable (vitamin C source) group?

A One serving is equivalent to:
    ¾ cup of citrus juice
    1½ cups of tomato or pineapple juice

½ grapefruit, cantaloupe, mango, papaya, or guava
½ cup strawberries
¾ cup of broccoli, brussel sprouts, cabbage, or cauliflower
½ cup green or red pepper

Q How much is one serving from the fruit and vegetable (vitamin A source) group?

A One serving is equivalent to:
   1 cup raw or ¾ cup cooked asparagus, broccoli, kale, spinach, carrots, winter squash, sweet potato, or yam
   1 medium apple
   1 medium banana

Q Why should I eat foods from the fruit and vegetable group?

A These foods provide you and your baby with vitamins A and C. These vitamins help heal wounds, resist infection, and provide for your night vision.

Q How much is one serving from the grain group?

A One serving is equivalent to:
   1 slice of bread
   1 roll, muffin, or biscuit
   1 six-inch flour tortilla
   2 corn tortillas
   5 saltine crackers
   2 graham crackers
   ¾ cup cooked cereal
   ¾ cup dry cereal
   ¾ cup rice, pasta, or grits
   1 tablespoon wheat germ

Q Why should I eat foods from the grain group?

A Whole-grain foods provide you and your baby with carbohydrates, B vitamins, iron, vitamin E, folic acid, and zinc. These foods are used for energy and to maintain a healthy nervous system.

Q Can I eat other foods that are not part of the groups listed?

A Of course. Other foods such as pastries, fats, and spices do make eating more enjoyable. They will provide you with some extra calories that you may need, or may not need, as the case may be. Limit your diet to a minimum of foods containing empty calories. Eat yogurt, ice milk, or puddings instead of chips or candy.

Q What is an example of a well-balanced diet?

A *Breakfast:*
    Orange juice
    Raisin bran
    One egg
    Whole-wheat toast, jam
    Milk
Snack:
    Banana
    Graham crackers
Lunch:
    Tuna sandwich
    Salad with tomatoes
    Fruit
    Milk

Snack:
    Oatmeal cookie
    Milk
Dinner:
    Cantaloupe
    Baked chicken
    Rice
    Peas
    Butter
    Milk
Snack:
    Ice milk

Q Why must I eat foods containing protein?

A Protein is necessary for the growth, development, and maintenance of your tissues and those of the fetus. Protein is made up of smaller units called amino acids. There are 20 different amino acids. Your body can produce 12 of them. The other eight are called the "essential" amino acids and must be eaten, because your body cannot manufacture them.

Q How much protein do I need to eat each day?

A The recommended amount of protein is about 80 grams per day.

Q *Which foods contain protein?*

A Protein is found in red meats, poultry, fish, and dairy products. These are complete protein foods, meaning they contain all the essential amino acids and can be eaten alone for an adequate source of protein. Many vegetables also contain protein, but each vegetable lacks one or more of the 8 essential amino acids. If you are a vegetarian, you must learn to combine your protein sources to take in all the essential amino acids.

Q *What amount of fluids should I drink each day?*

A You should drink about 8 to 10 glasses of fluids a day. Milk, fruit juices, soups, and water all count as liquids. So do carbonated beverages, but they are either diet (and contain aspartame) or nondiet (and contain quite a number of calories). Coffee and alcohol are liquids that should also be avoided.

Q *Should I limit my intake of salt (sodium)?*

A No. You may salt your foods to taste. There is no reason to restrict your salt intake. Salt is not the cause of toxemia, as was once believed. In fact, during pregnancy the requirement for sodium is increased. Of course, if you are experiencing annoying swelling of your ankles and feet, you may want to restrict your salt intake somewhat. Foods that contain a high-salt content are canned, packaged or frozen foods, fast foods, cold cuts, and pickles.

Q *Why should my diet contain fat?*

A Fats provide energy and are necessary for the absorption of the fat-soluble vitamins D, E, A and K, and calcium. There is an essential fat called linoleic acid that is not produced by your body, but that is necessary for the growth and maintenance of your tissues.

Q *How much fat should my diet contain?*

A Probably no more than 35% of your diet should be made up of fats. If you follow the diet guidelines above for eating animal proteins and grains, you will obtain a sufficient amount of fats.

Q *Why should my diet contain carbohydrates?*

A Carbohydrates contain B vitamins and vitamin C, and are also a quick source of energy. There are some forms of carbohydrates that are not nutritious, however. These are the refined sugars (white or brown sugar, honey, or molasses). They are a quick source of energy, calories, and weight gain. Try to eat foods containing complex carbohydrates instead, such as fruits, vegetables, grains, and cereals. These foods also contain a healthy amount of fiber which will prevent constipation.

Q *How much carbohydrate should my diet contain?*

A If you follow the meal plan suggestions above, you will eat the necessary amount of carbohydrates.

Q *Do pregnant women really have cravings for certain foods?*

A Yes. Sometimes a woman may crave citrus fruits because she actually needs more vitamin C, or a sweet because she has hypoglycemia (low blood sugar) at that time, usually in the middle of the night. Other food cravings may be more unusual; for instance, the practice of eating laundry starch, clay, or ice shavings from a freezer. This is called *pica* and may be due to severe iron deficiency, although this is not always the case. Some pregnant women in impoverished areas practice this commonly.

Q *Do some pregnant women have aversions to certain foods?*

A Yes. You may even develop a dislike to foods that you usually enjoy.

Q *Can I use artificial sweeteners during pregnancy?*

A There are now two principal types of artificial sweeteners on the market: saccharin and aspartame. Saccharin is known to cross the placenta, but has not been shown to cause an increase in miscarriages or birth defects, thus far. The same is true for aspartame. Aspartame is composed of two amino acids: phenylalanine and aspartic acid. Ingestion of phenylalanine is a problem for women who have a rare chemical birth defect which causes them to be unable to digest this amino acid. The disorder is called phenylketonuria (PKU), and the resulting accumulation of phenylalanine in the blood may cause mental retardation in the fetus. Potential problems are prevented by a diet low in phenylalanine during pregnancy in women with this disorder.

Until more is known about the effects of artificial sweeteners, limit your use of these chemicals during your pregnancy.

5 Health and Fitness Concerns

Q Do stress and anxiety affect the fetus?

A No. It is very common for pregnant women to experience mood swings throughout the day. You may become intensely angry or depressed and suffer from crying spells. Medical research has shown that stress and anxiety in no way affect the health and well-being of your fetus.

Q What can I do if I have or develop acne during pregnancy?

A First, increase the number of times you wash your face with soap and water. If the acne becomes severe, consult your doctor; he or she may recommend preparations containing benzoyl peroxide (i.e., Stridex or Clearasil) or cis-retinoic acid. These are safe if used in moderation. Do not use tetracycline or Accutane. (See medicines to avoid in Chapter 6).

Q What should I know about bathing during pregnancy?

A In general, baths during pregnancy are safe, with a few

precautions, however. Do not bathe in water warmer than 100°F. Hot water, especially in the early months of pregnancy, may cause congenital abnormalities such as neural tube defects in the fetus. Near the end of the second trimester and throughout the third trimester, make sure someone is home with you when you bathe. Remember your center of balance has changed due to your enlarging uterus, which makes slipping and falling an easy thing to do. Do not take a bath if your membranes have ruptured and you are leaking amniotic fluid; instead, take a shower before going to the hospital. A nice warm bath may help those of you who are having trouble falling asleep at night.

Q   *Can I sunbathe during my pregnancy?*

A   Yes, sunbathing is not harmful to your pregnancy. However, if you are prone to developing cholasma, this will intensify your mask of pregnancy.

Q   *Can I get a new pair of contact lenses during my pregnancy?*

A   No. There are temporary changes in the cornea of your eye, which can change your eyesight.

Q   *Why does my vision become blurred shortly after I put in my contact lenses?*

A   There is a change in the composition of your tears that may cause your contact lenses to become greasy.

Q   *Why are my contact lenses uncomfortable?*

A   Discomfort is caused by swelling of the cornea. This is most common near the end of pregnancy.

Q   *Can I douche when I am pregnant?*

A   I do not recommend routine douching, whether you are pregnant or not. However, some women cannot stand the excessive vaginal discharge occasionally present during pregnancy. If you must douche, do not use a bulb syringe; deaths from an air embolism have occurred. To prevent high pressure, the douche bag should not be placed more than 2 feet above your hips, and do not insert the nozzle more than 3 inches into your vagina.

Q *Does pregnancy make me more susceptible to tooth decay?*

A No, this is another myth. Pregnant women are just as likely as anyone else to develop tooth decay.

Q *Should I go to the dentist when I am pregnant?*

A Your routine dental checkups should continue when you are pregnant. If you have dental caries or need other procedures done, try waiting until the second trimester.

Q *Should I have dental x-rays taken during pregnancy?*

A If your dentist feels you need x-rays, have them done. The x-rays are directed away from your abdomen, which is shielded with a lead apron. There is little danger to your developing fetus.

Q *If I need dental work done, what kind of anesthesia is safe for my dentist to use?*

A The safest form of anesthesia for the pregnant patient is local anesthesia. Nitrous oxide, general anesthesia, and intravenous sedatives should be avoided.

Q *Should I use fluoride supplementation to prevent dental caries in my baby?*

A Preliminary studies have shown the safety and efficacy of fluoride supplementation during pregnancy, but more studies are needed before it can be recommended as a routine supplement.

Q *Can I have a permanent when I am pregnant?*

A Permanents are safe during pregnancy; however, some women experience thinning of their hair and may want to wait until after delivery for a new hairstyle.

Q *Can I dye my hair during pregnancy?*

A There have been no effects observed in the fetus from the application of hair dye.

Q *What kind of bra should I buy during pregnancy?*

A Cotton maternity bras offer the best support for your enlarging breasts. It is possible for you to change two or three cup sizes during your pregnancy. If your breasts are pendulous, you may want to wear a bra all the time. Buy your nursing bra a few weeks before your due date, and make sure it is one size larger than the bra you are wearing at the time.

Q *Can I use a hot tub or sauna during pregnancy?*

A Sure, but use the same precautions as with your bath—no temperature above 100°F.

Q *When should I take off my rings?*

A Not every pregnant woman has to remove her rings, but if one is starting to feel tight on your finger, take it off. If you wait too long, you will have to have it removed by the jeweler. A tight fitting ring can act like a tourniquet and stop the blood flow to your finger. If you are embarrassed to be seen pregnant and without your wedding ring, have your loved one buy a necklace to put your ring on!

Q *Can I cook with a microwave oven during my pregnancy?*

A It is safe to cook with a microwave oven during pregnancy. The microwaves are shielded by several safety features built into the oven. There is a possibility that you could be exposed to some microwaves from a leak in the door, but you would have to stand directly in front of the oven for several hours to receive any significant exposure. The energy of the waves becomes progressively weaker the farther you are from the oven, so even a leaking microwave could be used without any adverse consequence.

Q *Can I paint my baby's room if I am pregnant?*

A Yes. Most paints today are latex-based and are not harmful to your pregnancy. Years ago when paint was lead-based, there was a potential danger.

Q *Does loud noise affect the fetus?*

A Yes it does, but not adversely. A loud noise such as you would experience at a rock concert or at an airport is also heard by your fetus. The noise evokes a startled response in both you and your baby. The baby will react by moving and have an increased heart rate. This is a very healthy response to the noise. In fact, medical research is currently being done using sound to evoke this reaction and correlating it with fetal well-being.

Q *Can I use pesticides in the house when I am pregnant?*

A Pesticides can be used in your home during your pregnancy with no untoward side effects to you or your developing fetus if used sensibly. First, always have your partner or someone else in the house use pesticides. Second, if using a bomb, stay away from your home for at least eight hours after use. Third, keep the room well ventilated.

Q *Do house pets pose a threat if I have allergies to them?*

A If you had an allergy to a dog or a cat before you were pregnant you will continue to have an allergy to these pets when you are pregnant. The same precautions should be followed—avoid contact with them. You will experience the same symptoms, i.e., stuffed nose and teary eyes, but there will be no adverse effects to your fetus if this is the extent of your symptoms. If these symptoms are annoying enough, you will want to take an allergy medicine. As with all medications, they should be avoided if possible during pregnancy since they all have potentially adverse effects on your developing fetus.

TRAVEL

Q   *Can I travel in an airplane during my pregnancy?*

A   Yes, airplane travel is safe for you and your fetus during your pregnancy. If you suffer from motion sickness, there are medications you can take that are safe to use during pregnancy. However, try to delay your trip until the second trimester of your pregnancy.

Q   *Are there any special instructions for me if I am planning a long trip?*

A   Before you go on your trip, locate the nearest hospital and ask your doctor to recommend an obstetrician in that area should an emergency arise. If you will be gone for several weeks, take a copy of your prenatal records with you.

    If you are embarking on a long drive or plane ride, get up and move around every couple of hours to avoid swelling in your legs and feet.

Q   *Should I plan a trip near the end of my pregnancy?*

A   Your baby does not know your due date. He or she may come at any time near the end of pregnancy. You should not plan a trip after 34 weeks, if you want to deliver at the hospital of your choice, with the doctor of your choice.

Q   *If I am planning a trip abroad during my pregnancy, which immunizations should I receive and which ones should I avoid?*

A   The following is a summary of the recommendations of the American College of Obstetricians and Gynecologists (ACOG) for immunizations during pregnancy:

> *Cholera*—if needed for travel destination
> *Hepatitis A*—after exposure or if needed for travel destination
> *Hepatitis B*—safe if needed
> *Influenza*—safe if needed
> *Measles*—not safe
> *Mumps*—not safe

Plague—only if absolutely needed

Polio—not recommended, but can be taken if traveling to a high-risk area

Rabies—safe

Rubella—not safe

Tetanus-diptheria—safe if indicated

Typhoid—if needed for travel destination

Varicella (chicken pox)—varicella-zoster immune globulin is safe

Yellow fever—if needed for travel destination

Q *Should I wear seat belts when I am pregnant?*

A Yes. Beside being effective in preventing injury to yourself and your fetus, it is also the law in many states. You should wear both the lap belt and shoulder harness. The lap belt should be worn across the thighs, under the fetus, and against your hip bones. The shoulder harness should be worn above your uterus. You may also want to place a small pillow on your lap between your uterus and the steering wheel.

Q *Will the airport metal detector machines affect my baby?*

A No. The airport metal detector you walk through will not emit any form of harmful radiation to you or your fetus.

WORK

Q *Can I continue to work when I am pregnant?*

A Working is not harmful to you or your baby. Women who do not have physically strenuous jobs may continue their employment without difficulty. If you are concerned about potentially noxious vapors in your workplace, consult your doctor.

Q *Are video display terminals (VDTs) harmful to my pregnancy?*

A There is no evidence that exposure to VDTs causes either an increased incidence of miscarriages or birth defects.

Q When should I stop working?

A In general, you should stop working when you feel too tired to continue your usual work routine. Some women drive a long distance to and from work and may find commuting too tiresome. Many women will work up until the day they go into labor. The government allows *paid* maternity disability: 4 weeks before and 6 weeks after the birth of your baby, based on your due date. Take the time if you need it. Recently, the Supreme Court allowed an extended disability of 18 weeks for maternity leave after delivery. You cannot lose your job during this period; however, you will receive only 6 weeks of paid disability.

SEX

Q Can I have sexual intercourse during my pregnancy?

A Yes. You will not harm your pregnancy if you make love during this time. There are some conditions where sexual intercourse may be prohibited: a history of premature labor, threatened miscarriage, or premature rupture of membranes.

Q Can spotting of blood occur after having sex?

A This is a common occurrence. The cervix becomes very vascular and small blood vessels may break and bleed temporarily after sexual intercourse. There is no risk to your pregnancy.

Q Will my sex drive change during pregnancy?

A Some women feel more amorous, others less, and some women have the same desires as before they were pregnant. All of these are normal behavior.

Q Is it possible that having sex may feel uncomfortable?

A As your pregnancy progresses, the missionary position (man on top) may feel uncomfortable. Discuss and try different positions with your mate.

Q *Can my partner perform oral sex on me when I am pregnant?*

A Yes, this too is fine. However, do not have him blow into your vagina. Since the number of blood vessels formed in your vagina has increased, there is the possibility that air may enter your bloodstream and cause neurological problems or even death.

EXERCISE

Q *Is it safe—for both me and my baby—to exercise when I'm pregnant?*

A Medical research has recently pointed out that if you're physically fit before your pregnancy, you may continue to exercise during your pregnancy as long as you have no medical or obstetrical complications. Your main concern is that your fetus gets an adequate supply of oxygen. Mild aerobic activities such as walking, swimming, and relaxation exercises such as those taught at childbirth preparation classes are excellent. Follow the American College of Obstetricians and Gynecologists (ACOG) guidelines given at the end of this chapter.

Q *I'm in great shape. Can I continue to exercise at my present level?*

A Nature has its ways of curtailing your activities! During the first 13 weeks of pregnancy at least 50% of women experience nausea and vomiting. During the next 23 weeks, hormonal changes may cause fatigue and lack of motivation. Even if you don't suffer these changes, you should decrease your level of training to adapt to your weight gain, particularly from the 5th month on. The extra weight alone will make your normal workout more difficult.

Q *Is it safe to begin an exercise program once I become pregnant, if I've been sedentary up to this point?*

A Yes, you can begin an exercise program, but with some

limitations. For instance, now is not the time to strive to get into "world-class" shape. Once again, follow the ACOG guidelines.

Q *Must I stop exercising during my last month of pregnancy?*

A Not unless your doctor suggests you do so because of obstetrical complications. However, it would be advisable to cut back if you experience back problems, swelling of your extremities, lack of balance, or extreme fatigue or discomfort because of weight gain. If you experience none of the problems, then mild exercise is perfectly all right until you go into labor.

Q *How will I know if I am exercising too much?*

A If you follow the ACOG guidelines, eat a balanced diet but do not gain the prescribed 20 to 30 pounds, you may be exercising too much and too hard. I recommend that you consult your doctor to discuss modifying your exercise program and caloric intake. Physically fit women will lose their weight gain within the first 3 months after giving birth.

Q *What activities should I avoid when I'm pregnant?*

A Avoid sports such as snow and water skiing, horseback riding, and scuba diving. Your joints and ligaments become particularly lax during pregnancy, due to hormonal changes, and don't give you the support and stability necessary to safely perform some activities.

Q *Will exercise make my labor easier?*

A Unfortunately, no studies to date point this out. However, being in good shape will provide you with stamina, which is a plus when it comes to the strenuous task of delivering a baby.

ACOG GUIDELINES ON EXERCISE DURING PREGNANCY

During pregnancy and the postpartum period

1. Regular exercise (at least 3 times per week) is preferable to intermittent activity. Competitive activities should be discouraged.
2. Vigorous exercise should not be performed in hot, humid weather or during a period of febrile (feverish) illness.
3. Ballistic movements (jerky, bouncy motions) should be avoided. Exercise should be done on a wooden or a tightly carpeted surface to reduce shock and provide sure footing.
4. Deep flexion or extension of joints should be avoided because of connective tissue laxity. Avoid activities that require jumping, jarring motions, or rapid changes in direction.
5. Vigorous exercise should be preceded by a 5-minute period of muscular warm-up. This can include slow walking or stationary cycling with low resistance.
6. Vigorous exercise should be followed by a period of gradually declining activity that includes gentle, stationary stretching. Because connective tissue laxity increases the risk of joint injury, stretches should not be performed at maximum resistance.
7. Heart rate should be measured at peak activity. Do not exceed physician's established limits. In postpartum, stay within normal training heart rate range.
8. Care should be taken to gradually rise from the floor to avoid orthostatic hypotension (low blood pressure that occurs on rising to the erect position). Some form of activity involving the legs should be continued for a brief period.
9. Liquids should be taken liberally before and after exercise to prevent dehydration. If necessary, activity should be interrupted to replenish fluids.
10. Women who have led sedentary lifestyles should begin with physical activity of very low intensity (walking or marching in place) and advance gradually.
11. Activity should be stopped and the physician consulted if any unusual symptoms appear.

During pregnancy only

1. Maternal heart rate should not exceed 140 beats/minute.
2. Strenuous activities should not exceed 15 minutes in duration.
3. No exercises should be performed in the supine position after the 4th month of gestation.
4. Exercises that employ the Valsalva maneuver (holding your breath while bearing down as if you are having a bowel movement) should be avoided.
5. Caloric intake should be adequate to meet the extra energy needs of pregnancy as well as the exercise performed.
6. Maternal core temperature should not exceed 38.5°C (101.3°F).

6 *Drugs and Medications*

ALCOHOL

Q *Can I drink alcohol when I am pregnant?*

A The Surgeon General advises all pregnant women not to drink alcohol. This admonition is also found in the Bible: "Behold, thou shalt conceive, and bear a son, and now drink no wine or strong drink . . ." (Judges 13:7).

The placenta does not act as a barrier for alcohol. Any alcohol you drink will get into your developing baby's bloodstream and will be in the same concentration as in your own. So, if you have a drink, say a toast to your baby because he or she is drinking along with you. Before you have a drink, just think whether you would put even a little beer or wine in your baby's bottle.

Q *What are the effects to my pregnancy if I drink?*

A The risk of a miscarriage is twice as high if you drink only 1 ounce of absolute alcohol (AA) as rarely as twice a week. That is four glasses of wine per week. Women who drink more than 1.5 ounces of AA per day will have an increased risk of premature labor or postterm labor.

49

Q What are the effects of alcohol on my baby?

A The effects on your baby have been collectively termed the Fetal Alcohol Syndrome. These babies are born to chronic alcoholics, women who drink more than 6 drinks per day. These babies usually are mentally retarded, have poor coordination, are hyperactive, are smaller in both height and weight, and have characteristic facial features. In addition, a variety of other malformations have been reported in these babies.

Q Before I knew I was pregnant, I went on a few drinking binges. What will be the effect on my baby?

A No effect on the fetus from binge drinking in early pregnancy has been shown.

Q Before I knew I was pregnant, I would drink a glass of wine with dinner. How will this affect my baby?

A Currently, there is no evidence of adverse effects on the fetus with a daily alcohol consumption of 0.5 ounce AA per day. But two glasses of wine per day may cause abnormalities in up to 10% of babies.

Q How common is alcohol consumption during pregnancy?

A One study reported that up to 17% of pregnant women drink at least two drinks per week and that 4% drink daily.

CIGARETTES

Q Does smoking cigarettes cause an increased incidence of miscarriages?

A Yes, if you smoke, you are almost doubling your risk of miscarriage.

Q How does cigarette smoking cause problems during pregnancy?

A Cigarette smoke contains tar, nicotine, and carbon monoxide.

Tar coats your lungs and prevents oxygen from entering your bloodstream and your baby's. Carbon monoxide competes with oxygen for space on red blood cells, so less oxygen is available to the growing tissues of the fetus. Nicotine constricts blood vessels, causing less blood flow through the placenta. The result is that less nutrients pass to the fetus and it takes longer to clear out waste products.

Q What are the possible complications of smoking on my pregnancy?

A There is an increased risk of placenta previa, abruption, premature labor, and premature rupture of membranes.

Q What are the effects of cigarette smoking on my baby?

A Women who smoke have smaller babies. This is dose dependent. The more you smoke, the smaller your baby. The greatest decrease in weight is about 7 ounces. These children may also lag behind in learning ability by almost six months. There is also a much higher incidence of SIDS (Sudden Infant Death Syndrome) in pregnancies complicated by cigarette smoking.

ILLICIT DRUGS

Q What are the effects of marijuana smoking during pregnancy?

A The same effects as for cigarette smoking have been demonstrated for marijuana smoking during pregnancy. In addition, there seems to be an increased risk of prematurity, precipitous (fast) labor, and meconium passage (a sign of fetal distress).

Q What are the effects of smoking marijuana on my baby?

A No increased incidence of malformations in the fetus due to marijuana has been shown. However, babies born to women who are marijuana smokers have problems responding to environmental stimuli and may have tremors. These changes seem to resolve by the end of the first month of life.

Q What are the effects of cocaine use during pregnancy?

A Only small studies concerning the effects of cocaine use during pregnancy have been published, but with the rising use of cocaine in the United States, other larger studies will follow. Cocaine use has been linked to an increased incidence of abruptio placenta. Women who use cocaine are more likely to have first trimester miscarriages and premature labor.

Q What are the effects of cocaine use on my baby?

A Cocaine use has been linked to an increased incidence of SIDS. There also seem to be neurological changes in the newborn, a depressed response to environmental stimuli, and interactive behavior. The infants tend to be shorter, weigh less, and have smaller head circumferences. Cocaine has been found in breast milk 48 hours after its last use and at least one report has been published describing a cocaine overdose in an infant after being breastfed by a cocaine-abusing mother. More studies are needed to determine whether cocaine will produce birth defects in the fetus.

CAFFEINE

Q Can I drink coffee when I am pregnant?

A The effects of caffeine are inconclusive, but to be safe, limit your intake of coffee and other products that contain caffeine. One recent study demonstrated a twofold increase in miscarriages in women who drank 150 milligrams of caffeine per day (one strong cup or 3 to 4 weak cups of coffee). Caffeine is a stimulant and does cross the placenta. Tea also is a stimulant and, in addition, can prevent iron absorption when drunk with meals.

If you want to drink coffee, switch to a decaffeinated type or other coffee substitute. Remember that many sodas and over-the-counter medicines contain caffeine as well.

MEDICATIONS

Q Before I knew that I was pregnant I took a particular medication. What will this do to my baby?

A Exposure to a certain medicine or drug probably accounts for 2% to 3% of all birth defects. The fetus is most sensitive to a drug's effects during the period when its organs are developing. This takes place from the 31st to the 71st day after your last menstrual period. Any medicine or drug ingestion before this time has an all-or-none effect: either the fetus survives without birth defects or it does not survive.

Q Is it safe to take over-the-counter medicines when I am pregnant?

A A general rule is: Do not take any medicine, prescription or nonprescription, without the consent of your doctor. Another general rule is: Assume that all medicines are potentially harmful to your developing fetus.

A third general rule is: Only take a medicine whose benefit will far outweigh its potential risk to mother and fetus. Only your doctor can make that decision.

Despite the cautions to avoid drugs and the indiscriminate ingestion of medicine, recent surveys have found that the average pregnant woman takes up to 5 drugs or medicines during her pregnancy which contain 9 different pharmacologic agents. The most common are prenatal vitamins, iron supplements, antacids, antiemetics (antinausea medicines), analgesics, and antihistamines.

Q Should I take prenatal vitamins?

A If you eat three well-balanced meals a day, you will meet the requirements for vitamins and minerals required each day and not need a vitamin supplement. Unfortunately, many pregnant women for a variety of reasons (i.e., morning sickness, food cravings or aversions, "too busy," etc.) do not eat properly and may benefit from taking a prenatal vitamin. Prenatal vitamins are supplements and should not be used as a substitute for food.

Q Which prenatal vitamin should I take?

A Each doctor has his or her own preference of prescription or over-the-counter brands. Just remember to take your pill with food for better absorption. If you can't swallow pills, ask your doctor about taking children's chewable vitamins.

Q Should I take an iron supplement during pregnancy?

A Iron is another story. Even a well-balanced diet will not supply the increased requirements of iron needed during pregnancy, especially in the second half of pregnancy. It is recommended that all pregnant women take an iron supplement during pregnancy and after delivery if the baby will be breast-feeding.

   The iron pill should be taken with meals—for best absorption, with a meal containing vitamin C (for example, citrus fruits, tomatoes, or potatoes).

Q Which iron supplement should I take?

A Once again your doctor will suggest his favorite type. If you can't swallow the pill, ask your doctor about using iron in liquid form. Sustained-release iron preparations are expensive and offer no advantages. Iron combined with vitamin C and a laxative are also expensive. As an alternative, take your iron with orange juice and eat some dates or prunes for a snack later on in the day.

Q What are the possible side effects of taking iron?

A You will notice a change in your stools; they will become black and tarry. This is caused by the unabsorbed iron. Constipation or diarrhea, abdominal cramps, and nausea are other common complaints. Taking the iron supplements with meals may reduce these side effects. If you still are bothered, ask your doctor to switch you to an iron preparation containing a different salt (i.e., ferrous sulfate, ferrous gluconate, or ferrous fumarate). Do not take an antacid with your iron pill, since this will decrease its absorption.

Q *Before I became pregnant I took megavitamins. Can I continue to do so during my pregnancy?*

A The use of megavitamins can be dangerous whether you are pregnant or not. High doses of vitamin B_6 for prolonged periods of time may cause neurological problems, such as numbness or tingling in your hands and feet.

Vitamin A toxicity can cause fatigue, brittle nails, hair loss, scaly skin, joint pain, and abdominal pain. Your baby may be born with increased pressure in the spinal column and brain, bone decalcification, growth retardation, or possible abnormalities of the urinary tract system.

High doses of vitamin D for prolonged periods may cause nausea, vomiting, anorexia, hypertension, and calcium deposits in tissues other than your bones. Your baby could be born with mental retardation or a cleft palate.

Megadoses of vitamin C may cause kidney stones in you and scurvy in your baby.

As the old adage so aptly states: "Everything in moderation."

Q *Can I take aspirin when I am pregnant?*

A There is no evidence that aspirin causes birth defects. However, aspirin may cause bleeding in you and your newborn if taken within a week of delivery. If you want to take an aspirin for a headache, try lying down and relaxing first. Remember, too, aspirin is found in many over-the-counter cold and allergy medicines.

Q *Can I take acetaminophen (Tylenol, Datril, Panadol) during pregnancy?*

A There is no evidence that acetaminophen causes birth defects. It also is not toxic to the newborn. You may take acetaminophen for a fever over 100°F or other aches or pains under the direction of your doctor.

Q *Which medicines are known to have effects on the fetus?*

A Here is a list of medicines and their effects on the fetus:
   Accutane—birth defects
   Alcohol—birth defects

Coumadin—birth defects
DES—birth defects
Dilantin—birth defects
Methotrexate—birth defects
Methyl mercury—nerve damage, IUGR (intrauterine growth retardation)
Sulfa at term—jaundice
Testosterone—masculinization
Tetracycline—discoloration of teeth, decreased bone growth
Thalidomide—birth defects
Tobacco—prematurity, IUGR
Vaccinations (some)—birth defects
Vitamins (some in excess)—birth defects

X-RAYS

Q   *I had some x-rays performed before I realized that I was pregnant. What will happen to my baby?*

A   The risks of any birth defect to the fetus is extremely low due to diagnostic radiation exposure. Some studies have reported an increased likelihood of childhood leukemia in the offspring of women exposed to x-rays during pregnancy. This risk increases the number of leukemia cases from 2 per 6,000 to 3 per 6,000, a very small increase in risk compared to the risk of a newborn whose sibling has childhood leukemia (1 per 720).

Q   *Should I have x-ray studies when I am pregnant?*

A   The risk of birth defects to the fetus increases after a radiation exposure of from 5 to 10 rads. Most x-ray studies will not expose the fetus to this degree of risk, and, if ordered by your doctor, are necessary for your health and usually on an emergency basis. Of course, x-rays that can be avoided until after pregnancy should be delayed.

7 Special Tests

ALPHAFETOPROTEIN BLOOD TEST

Q *What is the alphafetoprotein (AFP) blood test?*

A This is a test that measures the amount of AFP in your circulation. All pregnant women have a certain normal amount of this substance circulating in their bloodstream. AFP is produced by the fetal liver and passes through the placenta into your circulatory system. An unusually high amount of AFP may indicate that your baby has a neural tube defect, such as spina bifida or anencephaly. A very low value may appear in women carrying a baby with Down's syndrome.

Q *When is this test taken?*

A This test is performed between the 15th and 20th week of pregnancy. The test is most accurate when done between the 16th and 18th week.

Q *If the AFP is high, does that mean that my baby has a neural tube defect?*

A No. The incidence of neural tube defects is 1 or 2 per 1,000 pregnancies. This test will be positive in 5 out of 100 pregnancies; therefore, if you have a positive test, you will have to undergo additional tests. It is possible that you are further along in your pregnancy or that you may be carrying twins. This test will detect all cases of anencephaly and approximately 80% of spina bifida.

Q *Will the AFP test always detect a Down's syndrome baby?*

A No, only about 20% will be detected.

Q *What additional tests will I take?*

A A repeat AFP blood test, an ultrasound, and an amniocentesis for confirming if your fetus has a neural tube defect or Down's syndrome.

Q *What is a neural tube defect?*

A This is a birth defect in the spine or skull of your fetus resulting in either anencephaly (the top of the skull is missing as is most of the brain) or spina bifida (part of the bones in the spine are not formed, allowing the spinal column to protrude out the back of the baby).

Q *Are these problems serious?*

A Babies born with anencephaly die within 48 hours of birth. There are varying degrees of spina bifida, depending on the size of the opening, where the defect is located, and if the nerves are covered with skin. Most babies born with spina bifida are paralyzed or very weak from the waist down, cannot control their bladder or bowels, are mentally retarded, and may eventually develop hydrocephalus (water on the brain).

Q *If I've had one child with a neural tube defect, what are my chances of having another?*

A About 5%.

ULTRASOUND

Q *What is an ultrasound?*

A An ultrasound is a machine that uses high-frequency sound waves (that cannot be heard) to produce a picture of the fetus. These sound waves are produced by a transducer, a hand-held instrument which is placed over your abdomen. The waves bounce off the organs and tissues of the fetus and placenta and are picked up by the transducer and translated into a picture by a computer onto a video screen. With the ultrasound, many malformations can be detected, but not all. The age of the fetus can be ascertained by measuring the fetal head, abdomen, and thigh bone, the position and age of the placenta can be determined, the amount of amniotic fluid can be measured, and the sex of your baby and the number of fetuses may be seen. The image of your baby may be hard for you to visualize, so ask your doctor to point out what he or she sees. The doptone the doctor uses to listen to the fetal heart tones and the external fetal monitor used during labor also employ ultrasound waves. Ultrasound is not known to harm you or the fetus.

Q *Is it necessary to perform an ultrasound during my pregnancy?*

A Some doctors perform one or two ultrasounds routinely during a pregnancy, other doctors only for specific indications. Ask your doctor about his or her practice.

Q *What are some indications for an ultrasound exam?*

A
- Vaginal bleeding in the first trimester—to determine if the fetus is alive
- Vaginal bleeding in the second or third trimester—to determine if the fetus is alive and to locate the placenta (in order to rule out placenta previa)
- To check for fetal life during any trimester
- To determine the gestational age of the fetus if you are unsure of your LMP or the size of your pregnancy does not equal the gestational age
- If you are having an amniocentesis
- If twins are suspected

- If intrauterine growth retardation is suspected
- If congenital abnormalities are suspected
- If a breech presentation is suspected
- To evaluate the quantity of amniotic fluid
- To perform a biophysical profile if indicated
- To determine fetal size
- To evaluate fetal maturity
- To evaluate a pelvic mass during pregnancy, such as fibroid or ovarian cyst

Q **What is a biophysical profile?**

A This screening test employs the use of both the external fetal monitor and the ultrasound machine. First, a nonstress test is performed and is followed by an ultrasound exam. During the ultrasound, your doctor will look at the amount of amniotic fluid, fetal muscle tone, breathing movements, and limb or body movement. Each of the categories receives a score of 0 (abnormal) or 2 (normal). A low score may indicate the need for delivery, especially if the pregnancy is near term.

AMNIOCENTESIS

Q **What is amniocentesis?**

A Amniocentesis is the removal of amniotic fluid with a needle that goes through your abdomen and into your uterus.

Q **How is it performed?**

A First, an ultrasound is done to determine that there is an adequate amount of amniotic fluid to remove and an area free of placenta and baby where the needle can be inserted. Your abdomen is then cleaned and a local anesthetic is injected into your skin at the site to be used by the amniocentesis needle. Then, using the ultrasound, a long needle is guided into your uterus (avoiding the placenta and your fetus), and a small amount of amniotic fluid is removed.

Q **Why is amniocentesis performed?**

A This test can be done to determine the presence or absence of chromosomal disorders (i.e., Down's syndrome, Tay-Sach's disease, hemophilia), fetal lung maturity, a neural tube defect, severity of Rh disease, or intrauterine infection.

Q *When is an amniocentesis performed to detect genetic abnormalities?*

A A genetic amniocentesis is performed between the 15th and 17th week of your pregnancy.

Q *What are the complications of amniocentesis?*

A The risk of complications is low, less than 1%. You could experience temporary cramping, scant bleeding, or leak amniotic fluid, which are self-limiting and do not need treatment. Severe bleeding, infection, miscarriage, and death have occurred but are extremely rare events. If you are Rh negative, you should have an injection of Rh immune globulin after the procedure. With the use of ultrasound, the fetus, cord, or placenta are rarely stuck by the needle. If performed near term, rupture of membranes or the initiation of labor rarely occurs. As with any procedure, the benefits should outweigh the risks.

GROUP B *B*-STREPTOCOCCUS

Q *What is the group B B-streptococcus test?*

A This tests for the presence of the *B*-strep bacteria in your vagina and rectum. It is a simple and rapid test to perform. The doctor will place a Q-tip at the opening of your vagina and another at the opening of your rectum for culture. This test may be performed at an office visit during the early part of the third trimester.

Q *Why is this test done?*

A Thirty percent of women (pregnant or nonpregnant) harbor this bacteria. If you do, you don't know it, and there usually are no signs of infection. Babies born to mothers with *B*-strep may develop a severe pneumonia or meningitis (1 in 300). Premature babies are at greatest risk (1 in 150). There are approximately 15,000 babies born each year who become infected with group B *B*-streptococcus.

Q *How can infection in my baby be prevented?*

A Prevention is simple. Ampicillin given through your I.V. during labor will prevent infection of your baby.

HEPATITIS B VIRUS SCREENING

Q *What is the hepatitis B virus screening test?*

A This test screens for women who are chronic carriers of the hepatitis B virus. Many women who have become infected with this virus are unaware that they have had this infection or are carriers. This blood test may be done at your first prenatal visit.

Q *Who should get screened for hepatitis B virus?*

A This test is recommended for only high-risk individuals such as:
- Women of Asian, Pacific Island, or Eskimo descent
- Women born in Haiti or sub-Saharan Africa
- Health care workers handling blood
- Women with a history of liver disease
- Women with a history of intravenous illicit drug use
- Staff at institutions for the mentally retarded
- Women with a history of blood transfusions
- Women with a sexual partner who has had hepatitis B

Q *Why is it important to have this test?*

A Infants born to mothers with a positive hepatitis B test may become infected with the virus. About 25% of these babies could become chronic carriers and develop cirrhosis (major damage) or cancer of the liver. If your doctor knows that you have chronic hepatitis he or she can alert your pediatrician. Your baby will then receive a series of injections that will greatly reduce the chance of a hepatitis B virus infection and its effects.

DIABETES SCREENING

Q *What is the diabetes screening test?*

A This is a blood test performed between the 24th and 28th week of your pregnancy. One hour before this test you will be asked to drink 5 ounces of sugar water. This test, if positive, is followed by a longer 3-hour oral glucose tolerance test to determine if you have diabetes. If you do have an abnormal test result, you may require treatment with diet and/or insulin. If all pregnant patients are screened, approximately 3% will have gestational diabetes (diabetes of pregnancy, see diabetes in Chapter 9).

TOXOPLASMOSIS

Q *What is toxoplasmosis?*

A This is an infection caused by a one-celled organism called toxoplasmosis gondii. In up to 90% of cases during pregnancy the infection is asymptomatic. The risk of contracting this disease during pregnancy is rare, 2 to 7 per 1,000 pregnant women annually. The infection can be transmitted to your fetus only if you become infected during your pregnancy. If you have a toxoplasmosis infection before becoming pregnant you cannot transmit it to your fetus.

Q *Is there a test I can take to find out if I have toxoplasmosis?*

A Yes. It is a blood test that will tell you if you have a recent or past infection. If you own a cat or eat exotic foods, such as steak tartare or carpaccio, ask your doctor to perform this test.

Q *How can I become infected with toxoplasmosis?*

A By eating undercooked or raw meat infected with toxoplasmosis or by coming into contact with infected cat feces. In general, only cats that are allowed outdoors acquire this disease.

Q If I become infected with toxoplasmosis during my pregnancy, will my baby become infected?

A The risk of infection to the fetus depends on the stage of your pregnancy: 5% in the first trimester; 30% in the second trimester; 60% in the third trimester.

Q If my baby becomes infected, what will happen?

A Most congenital infections are mild or have no apparent effect, especially if contracted late in pregnancy where almost 90% of babies appear to be normal. However, if your infection occurs in the first trimester and the fetus becomes infected as well, up to 75% may develop severe problems, such as blindness, hydrocephalus, or mental retardation.

ELECTRONIC FETAL MONITORING

Q What is electronic fetal monitoring?

A Electronic fetal monitoring is performed by a machine that records the fetal heartbeat and your uterine contractions. It can do this by internal or external attachment devices. External fetal monitoring uses an ultrasound device like the doptone instrument to pick up the fetal heart rate and a pressure monitor placed on your abdomen to detect uterine contractions. The machine then records this information on a moving strip of paper. Internal monitoring can be done only when your cervix is dilated and your membranes have ruptured, either spontaneously or by your doctor. An electrode (a small, thin wire shaped like a corkscrew) is attached to your baby's scalp for a more accurate recording of the heart rate and a thin water-filled tube is placed in your uterus through the cervix to record the exact strength of your contractions. Many doctors use external fetal monitors routinely during labor.

Q When are internal monitors used during labor?

A The internal fetal monitors are used whenever the fetal heart rate tracing looks abnormal on the external monitors. It is also used if there is meconium in the amniotic fluid, if pitocin augmentation of labor is needed, or an epidural anesthetic is used for pain during labor.

Q *Will my labor be monitored?*

A This is a question that can only be answered by your doctor. It has become routine in most hospitals.

Q *Can I move in bed while I am being monitored?*

A Of course you can. If the external monitor is used, your nurse will readjust the instruments if need be; the internal monitors are not affected by movement.

Q *Can the fetal monitor help me and my coach during labor?*

A Yes. Your coach can see when a contraction is starting and inform you when the peak of the contraction is occurring. This may be a great help in modifying your relaxation and breathing techniques.

Q *Can my baby get an electric shock from the internal scalp electrode?*

A No. Electric current does not pass along this line.

NONSTRESS TEST

Q *What is a nonstress test?*

A The nonstress test is a test of fetal well-being. The external fetal monitor is utilized for this test. The fetal heart rate will be recorded and you will be asked to mark down when you feel your baby move. A good or reactive test will demonstrate variability of the heart rate and accelerations of the heart rate during fetal movement. This test may be done in the office or hospital anytime after the 30th week. The test usually takes no more than 45 minutes to perform. The test may be performed at weekly or twice weekly intervals until delivery.

Q *What are some indications for doing a nonstress test?*

A
- Decreased fetal movement
- Postterm pregnancy
- Intrauterine growth retardation (small baby)
- Toxemia
- Maternal diabetes mellitus

Q What happens if I have a nonreactive nonstress test?

A If your pregnancy is close to term and your cervix is ready (ripe) for delivery, you will undergo an induction of labor (see page 128). If your pregnancy is far from term, other tests will be performed to confirm this result.

NIPPLE STIMULATION TEST

Q What is a nipple stimulation test?

A This is another screening test of fetal well-being. This test may be used as the first test employed or as a backup test after a nonreactive nonstress test. The external fetal monitor is used again, but this time both the ultrasound and pressure transducers are used. You will be asked to roll your nipple between your fingers. This will cause release of oxytocin, a hormone from the pituitary gland, which will stimulate mild uterine contractions. The fetal heart rate will be observed during these contractions for signs of stress. If none is observed, fetal well-being is documented. This test also takes about 45 minutes and may be repeated weekly or twice weekly. Premature labor has not been a common complication of this test.

CHORIONIC VILLUS SAMPLING (CVS)

Q What is chorionic villus sampling (CVS)?

A CVS is a new technique used to remove a small piece of growing placental tissue (chorionic villi) from the uterus. The tissue is then grown in a culture and examined for chromosomal abnormalities.

Q Who might want CVS?

A The most common pregnant patient undergoing CVS is one who will be 35 years old by the time of her delivery. Other indications, as with amniocentesis, are parents with a child with trisomy (Down's syndrome), parents that are carriers of an autosomal recessive disorder (Tay-Sachs disease), or carriers of a sex-linked disorder (hemophilia). CVS cannot detect pregnancies complicated with neural tube defects, so parents who have had a previous child with this disorder should have an amniocentesis.

Q When is CVS performed?

A This test is done between the 9th and 11th weeks of pregnancy.

Q Is anything done before I have CVS?

A You will have an ultrasound exam to confirm the length of your pregnancy. A cervical culture for gonorrhea and chlamydia will be taken. You will also attend a genetics counseling session.

Q How is CVS performed?

A Using ultrasound for guidance, a thin catheter (tube) is placed through the cervix and into the uterus. The catheter is moved next to the growing placenta and gentle suction is used to remove a small sample of tissue. An adequate amount of tissue is obtained 98% of the time. This procedure may be done in an office setting and is as uncomfortable as a pelvic exam with a speculum.

Q How long does it take to get the results of the CVS?

A Most results are obtained within 2 weeks.

Q How safe is CVS?

A The major complication of CVS is miscarriage. This occurs in 3% of mothers after the procedure. The risk of a miscarriage after a genetic amniocentesis is 0.5%. There have been no reports of premature labor or fetal anomalies resulting from CVS.

Q What are the advantages of CVS over amniocentesis?

A The major advantage is the timing of the procedure; it is performed in the first trimester. Therefore, if a lethal or severe problem is identified with your fetus, a termination of pregnancy, if desired, can be performed during the first trimester. The abortion performed during the first trimester is safer than that performed after amniocentesis in the second trimester.

Q *Where is CVS performed?*

A At the present time, CVS is being done in a few research centers in the United States. Ask your doctor for the closest center in your area, if you wish to undergo this procedure.

FETAL MOVEMENT TEST

Q *What is the fetal movement test?*

A This is a test that can be performed by you at home anytime after the 28th week of your pregnancy. Doctors have found that if the fetus moves at least ten times in a 12-hour period, the fetus is healthy. Other doctors have found that three movements in 1 hour correlate with a healthy baby.

Q *Is the fetus more active at night?*

A No. The fetus has its own sleep-wake cycle. For example, near term the fetus usually is active for about 35 minutes, then is inactive or sleeps for about 20 minutes. You probably notice the movements more often at night in bed, because you are not distracted by normal daytime activities.

Q *Is the fetus more active after I eat a meal?*

A There is no difference in fetal movements before, after, or during a meal.

Q *What can decrease fetal movements?*

A The use of alcohol, cigarettes, sedatives, and narcotics all decrease the movement of your fetus.

Q *Why count fetal movements?*

A If you are worried about the health of your fetus, this is an inexpensive, simple, and accurate method to reassure yourself that your fetus is well.

Q *How do you count fetal movements?*

A Begin counting the baby's movements as soon as you wake up in the morning.

Count ten individual times the baby moves. The movement can be either a kick, a swish, a turn, or a flip.

Record the time of the 10th movement every day.

Call the doctor if any of the following occurs:

- You do not feel the 10th movement by 6 P.M.
- The baby has not moved all day
- It is taking longer each day to get the 10th movement
  Remember:
- The baby may move all 10 times in ½ hour.
- The baby may take 8 hours to move 10 times.
- You should know what is characteristic of your baby so that you can tell your doctor or nurse when something different is happening.

Again, if the baby has not moved 10 times by 6 P.M., *call your doctor!*

8 Obstetrical Complications of Pregnancy

MISCARRIAGE

Q *What is a miscarriage?*

A Miscarriage or spontaneous abortion is the termination of pregnancy on or before 20 weeks. Most miscarriages occur in the first trimester, usually before the end of the 8th week.

Q *How common are miscarriages?*

A About 12% to 15% of pregnancies end by miscarriage.

Q *What are the causes?*

A At least 60% of miscarriages are due to a chromosomally abnormal embryo. In fact, 50% of miscarriages are "blighted ovums" or pregnancies where the embryo has died and only the placenta develops. The other 10% consist of genetic problems such as Down's syndrome. The abnormal genetic material may come from the egg or the sperm. A congenitally abnormal uterus or a uterus with a fibroid tumor may cause a miscarriage in the second trimester.

Q *Can emotional stress—anxiety, fear, anger, or fright— cause a miscarriage?*

A There is no evidence that emotions can cause a miscarriage.

Q *What are the risk factors?*

A Smoking, moderate drinking (alcohol), caffeine, two previous miscarriages, and poor nutrition increase your risk for an early miscarriage.

Q *What are the warning signs?*

A A subtle sign is the loss of the symptoms of pregnancy. You don't feel tired, your breasts aren't sore, and your nausea, if present, has disappeared. Most miscarriages occur 1 to 3 weeks after the death of the fetus. Vaginal spotting or bleeding is a danger sign. This occurs in about 25% of pregnancies, but at most one-half of these cases actually end in miscarriage. The bleeding may be due to implantation of the embryo, broken blood vessels in the cervix, or a bleeding cervical polyp. Cramping usually does not occur until you are actually having a miscarriage.

Q *If I am experiencing vaginal bleeding in the first trimester, how do I know if I am having a miscarriage?*

A You don't know. This condition is called a threatened abortion. A general rule of thumb is if you still have symptoms of pregnancy, you probably still have a good pregnancy. If you are having spotting, your doctor may ask you to stay in bed and refrain from sexual intercourse for 24 to 48 hours. If your bleeding is heavier, you may be asked to undergo a pelvic examination to assess the size of your uterus or an ultrasound examination to look for signs of fetal activity. Initially, the doctor will look at your cervix. If the cervix is dilated, you are having a miscarriage; if not, a pelvic exam will be done to measure the size of your uterus. A uterus smaller than indicated by the length of your pregnancy will lead to an ultrasound exam to find the cause of this discrepancy. The fetal heart may be seen pumping by 6 weeks. If you are less than 6 weeks pregnant, a blood test called a quantitative (number value) Beta HCG (human chorionic gonadotropin) may be drawn every other day to assess the growth of the pregnancy. The *B*-HCG is a hormone made by the placenta and its value almost doubles every 2 days; therefore, a healthy early pregnancy can be detected by this test. The combination of ultrasound, pelvic exam, and quantitative *B*-HCG can also be used to diagnose an ectopic pregnancy (discussed later in this chapter).

Q *What happens to me if I do have a miscarriage?*

A This depends on the age of your pregnancy. If the pregnancy is less than 7 weeks, you may have a complete miscarriage; if greater than 7 weeks, more often than not the miscarriage is incomplete, the cervix is dilated, bleeding is brisk, and there is still part of the placenta inside your uterus. You will need a D&C.

Q *What is a D&C?*

A D&C stands for dilatation and curettage. Most often, the cervix is already dilated, so just the uterine curettage is necessary. Curettage is cleaning out the uterus. A plastic suction device is used. General or local anesthesia may be used for the procedure. The procedure takes less than 20 minutes and can be done in the doctor's office or in the hospital on a same-day basis.

Q *What can I do after the D&C?*

A Physical recovery after a miscarriage and D&C occurs very quickly. Your only restrictions will be to avoid sexual inter-course, the use of tampons, or douching for a period of 2 weeks. If your blood loss was not excessive, and it usually isn't, you may resume your normal daily activities the following day. Emotionally, however, you may not feel up to doing anything for a period of time. You will be grieving and will go through the process of mourning.

Q *How long can I expect to have vaginal spotting?*

A You may have scant vaginal bleeding for up to 2 weeks after a miscarriage. Your doctor may give you a medicine called methergine, to take for a day or two. Methergine makes your uterus contract. This will slow down the bleeding, but may cause you to feel uterine cramping.

Q *How soon can we try again to conceive?*

A There is no harm in trying to conceive as soon as you want to after a miscarriage.

Q *If I have had a miscarriage, how common is another one with my next pregnancy?*

A If the first miscarriage was due to chromosomal abnormality of the fetus, your chance of a second miscarriage is only 7%. If not, it may be due to a problem with your uterus, increasing your chance of a miscarriage to 24%.

Q *If I have had two miscarriages in a row, what are my chances of having another?*

A About 24%. The risk does not increase after the second miscarriage.

Q *If I have Rh negative blood, do I need Rh immune globulin?*

A Yes, you should get an injection of RhoGam within 72 hours of your miscarriage.

ABRUPTIO PLACENTA

Q *What is abruptio placenta?*

A Abruptio placenta is the premature separation of the placenta after the 20th week of pregnancy and before the baby has been delivered. This condition may be dangerous, because when the placenta detaches, the fetus loses some of its supply of blood and oxygen. Since the site where the placenta attaches is filled with blood vessels, detachment causes bleeding from this area in the uterus.

Q *What are the signs of abruption?*

A Heavy vaginal bleeding with severe abdominal pain with or without regular uterine contractions occurs with an advanced stage of placental detachment. The amount of bleeding and degree of pain is proportional to the amount of placental separation. In about 33% of cases, the detachment is small and only a bit of spotting may be noted.

Q *How common is abruptio placenta?*

A Placental abruption occurs in about 1 in 250 pregnancies. About 50% of these occur before the 36th week of pregnancy.

Q *Who is at risk for getting an abruption?*

A Abruption occurs more frequently in pregnancies complicated by chronic hypertension, toxemia, diabetes, twins, and poor nutrition. Abdominal trauma causing an abruption is rare.

Q *What happens if I have an abruption?*

A This, of course, depends on the degree of placental attachment. If only a small area detaches, your bleeding will have been transient, and watchful waiting with decreased activity will be required. If a larger area detaches and bleeding and labor ensue, an early delivery will result. If bleeding is very heavy and signs of fetal distress are noted, an emergency cesarean section may be performed.

PLACENTA PREVIA

Q *What is placenta previa?*

A The placenta has implanted low in the uterus and has grown near or over the internal opening of the cervix.

Q *Why is this condition a problem?*

A As you approach the end of your pregnancy, the lower segment of the uterus begins to thin out and the cervix may begin to efface and dilate causing part of the placenta to detach from this area and resulting in "painless vaginal bleeding," the cardinal sign of placenta previa.

Q *How common is placenta previa?*

A The incidence of placenta previa is 1 in 200 pregnancies (0.5%). It is more common in women who have already had children: only 10% occur in first, full-term pregnancies. Women having more than 4 pregnancies have a 1 in 20 chance of having placenta previa with their next pregnancy.

Q *What causes placenta previa?*

A The cause is unknown, but we do know some of the risk factors. As stated above, a prior pregnancy increases the likelihood for placenta previa. The incidence is doubled in twins, probably because of the increased size of the placenta. The incidence is tripled in a pregnancy following a cesarean section with a low transverse uterine scar.

Q *If I experience painless vaginal bleeding, what should I do?*

A Call your doctor immediately. The first episode of bleeding (there can be more than one) is usually sudden in onset, painless, and profuse. Your clothes will become soaked with bright-red blood and seeing this may cause you to faint. The blood loss, which may only be scant spotting or as much as a cup or two of blood, however, rarely causes shock, and death is extremely rare.

Q *If I have a placenta previa, when is the most common time for bleeding to occur?*

A The first bleeding episode usually occurs around the 30th week of your pregnancy.

Q *What will the doctor do?*

A The doctor will meet you at his or her office or in the hospital, depending on the amount of blood loss, whether you are still bleeding, and the time of day. Usually the first episode of bleeding, although copious, is short lived. An ultrasound examination will be performed to confirm or rule out a placenta previa. Ultrasound is accurate in 97% of cases. If you do have a placenta previa, management will depend on the maturity of your fetus. Usually your doctor will try to delay birth of your baby until the 37th week.

Q If my pregnancy is less than 37 weeks, what will happen next?

A You will be hospitalized for about 3 days, confined to bed for 48 hours, and then allowed to walk to the bathroom on the 3rd day. You will have an I.V. and blood tests will be performed to check for anemia and type and crossmatch of blood. You will need a blood transfusion if you are very anemic. You will be discharged to home on bedrest only if you have stopped bleeding, if you live near the hospital, and if someone is with you at all times who can bring you back to the hospital if bleeding recurs. The doctor may ask you to have a blood test every 72 hours for crossmatching, so if profuse bleeding does recur, blood is immediately available for transfusion. In at least 75% of cases of placenta previa, the pregnancy will continue to the 36th week.

Q What happens if the bleeding continues?

A You will be taken to the operating room and the doctor will do a pelvic exam. If the diagnosis of placenta previa is confirmed, you will have a cesarean section, usually under general anesthesia.

Q If my pregnancy is 37 weeks or more, how will the doctor deliver my baby?

A The doctor will perform a cesarean section. If done on an elective basis, you will have your choice of anesthesia.

Q An ultrasound examination performed at 18 weeks showed a placenta previa. Does that mean I will need a cesarean section?

A Probably not. It has been shown that the incidence of placenta previa is much greater in the first and second trimesters than at term. During your advancing pregnancy, the placenta "migrates" away from the lower portion of the uterus, so your chances of having a placenta previa at term are only 1 in 20, as is your risk of cesarean section for this problem.

Q *What are the risks to my baby?*

A The perinatal mortality rate is about 15% to 20%, about ten times greater than in a normal pregnancy. The main causes of death are prematurity, lack of oxygen to the fetus, and congenital abnormalities.

TOXEMIA

Q *What is toxemia of pregnancy?*

A Toxemia or preeclampsia or pregnancy induced hypertension (PIH) is a disorder that usually occurs in the third trimester. There is a sudden increase in weight due to water retention, high blood pressure, and/or the appearance of protein in the urine. Most cases are mild.

Q *What is the cause?*

A There are many theories, but the causes of this disease are still undetermined.

Q *How common is toxemia?*

A Nationwide, it is about 5%. It occurs in about 15% of pregnant patients attending a teaching hospital and 1% to 2% of pregnant patients seen by an obstetrician in a private setting.

Q *What are the risk factors?*

A Being pregnant for the first time is a risk factor, since 65% of toxemia occurs in first-time mothers. It is even more common if the mother-to-be is under the age of 17, or 35 or older. Toxemia is 3 times as common with a twin pregnancy. It is also more common in women with previous hypertension. There seems to be a familial tendency toward the development of toxemia. Poor nutrition and dietary habits increase the risk.

Q *How can toxemia be prevented?*

A Begin your prenatal care early and don't cancel your appointments. Eat a well-balanced diet.

Q *What is the treatment for mild toxemia?*

A If you are near the end of your pregnancy and your cervix is ripe, the treatment is labor and delivery. If you develop toxemia early in the third timester, the treatment is bedrest throughout most of the day and a diet high in protein. You will be seen by the doctor twice a week and will undergo a nonstress or nipple stimulation test at least weekly. Delivery by induction will occur when your cervix is ripe, or if the severity of the disease progresses, induction and/or cesarean section will be performed regardless of the state of your cervix.

Q *What are the complications of toxemia?*

A The major complication of mild toxemia is the progression to the severe form with the development of blood clotting problems, liver dysfunction, convulsions, and very rarely death. Severe toxemia requires hospitalization to stabilize your condition.

Q *Are there warning signs for severe toxemia?*

A Yes. Headache, blurry vision, swelling of hands and face, and pain under the right side of your rib cage. Notify you doctor immediately if any of these symptoms occur.

Q *Is toxemia dangerous to my baby?*

A Toxemia causes the placenta to work less effectively, thus providing less nourishment to the fetus. As a result, the fetus will not grow as well, and in severe cases, may actually be in distress.

Q *Are there any special precautions during labor?*

A You will have an I.V. and internal fetal monitoring. You will receive magnesium sulfate, a drug that prevents convulsions, through your I.V.

Q What happens after delivery?

A Delivery is the cure for toxemia. Your blood pressure usually returns to normal and the increased water weight begins to disappear within 48 hours.

Q If I developed toxemia with my first pregnancy, will I have it again with my next pregnancy?

A Probably not. The recurrence of toxemia in subsequent pregnancies is rare.

BREECH

Q How common is a breech presentation?

A At term, the incidence of breech presentation is about 3%; however, it is much more common early in your pregnancy. About 33% are breech at 20 weeks, 25% at 28 weeks, and 9% at 36 weeks.

Q If I have a breech baby past 36 weeks, will it turn?

A From 37 weeks on, the chances of spontaneous turning are rare. However, if desired, you may ask your doctor about external cephalic version.

Q What is external cephalic version?

A This is the turning of the fetus from the breech to the vertex (head down) position. It is performed in the hospital after an ultrasound exam to confirm fetal position and well-being. You will have an I.V., and ritodrine—a uterine muscle relaxant—will be used. The doctor, usually a perinatologist, will then turn your baby. This may take up to 10 minutes and is only mildly uncomfortable. The success rate for turning is as high as 75%. The procedure is safe, with an extremely low incidence of complications.

Q If I don't want external cephalic version, how will my baby be delivered?

A Most doctors will perform a cesarean section. The chance of a negative outcome for your baby, both in terms of birth trauma and death, is higher with a vaginal delivery. There are doctors who will perform a vaginal delivery in selected cases.

Rh DISEASE

Q *What is the Rh factor?*

A The Rh factor is a protein found on the outside of the red blood cells of all rhesus monkeys. It is also found on most human blood cells. If it is on your red blood cells, you are Rh positive; if not found on your red blood cells, you have Rh negative blood.

Q *How does the Rh factor cause a problem?*

A The problem occurs when an Rh negative woman comes into contact with the Rh factor. Since this is a foreign substance to the bloodstream, your immune system will make antibodies to attack it. During pregnancy, especially in the last trimester, some of the fetal red blood cells may cross the placenta and enter your bloodstream. When this occurs during your first pregnancy, you will become sensitized, and you will form antibodies. Usually, not enough antibodies form to cause a problem. These antibodies, however, are permanent. During a second pregnancy, as soon as a small amount of Rh positive fetal red blood cells enter your circulation, you start to make these Rh antibodies again and this time in larger amounts. These antibodies are small enough to pass through the placenta and enter the bloodstream of your fetus. Once there, the antibodies attack the Rh positive red blood cells and cause them to burst. This is called *hemolysis*. The fetus becomes anemic and jaundiced. Jaundice is a yellow appearance of the skin due to the breakdown products of hemoglobin from the broken blood cells.

Q *How common is Rh incompatibility?*

A About 13% of pregnancies have Rh incompatibility.

Q *Are there other ways for Rh sensitization to occur?*

A Yes, if incompatibility exists, Rh sensitization may occur after a miscarriage, induced abortion, ectopic (tubal) pregnancy, or amniocentesis.

Q *How are Rh sensitization and hemolytic disease of the newborn prevented?*

A Rh disease can be prevented by a vaccine of Rh immune globulin. The vaccine contains antibodies which will bind to any fetal red blood cell present in your circulation and therefore prevent your immune system from becoming stimulated to form antibodies of its own. These antibodies last only 3 months, so repeated injections may be given.

Q *When should I receive Rh immune globulin?*

A It has been shown that receiving Rh immune globulin at 28 weeks and within 72 hours of delivery will prevent sensitization in 99.2% of Rh negative mothers. The vaccine should also be administered after a miscarriage, ectopic pregnancy, and amniocentesis.

Q *If I did not receive Rh immune globulin, what are my chances of becoming sensitized?*

A • 11% after a delivery
• 5% after amniocentesis
• 5% after an ectopic pregnancy
• 3% after a miscarriage or induced abortion

Q *How is Rh immune globulin administered?*

A The vaccine is injected into the muscle of the arm, thigh, or buttock. The only side effects are muscle soreness at the injection site or a low-grade fever. The vaccine is safe for the fetus.

Q *If I have a positive Rh titer, can I still receive the Rh immune globulin?*

A No. This means that you are already sensitized; you are producing Rh antibodies.

Q *What happens if I am Rh sensitized?*

A The doctor will discover Rh antibodies when the Rh titer is drawn. If a large amount of antibodies is present, an amniocentesis will be performed. Analysis of the amniotic fluid for bilirubin—a breakdown product of hemoglobin—will determine the severity of the effects on your baby. Ultrasound can also be used to follow the course of the hemolytic disease. The effects can range from mild to severe anemia in the fetus. With mild cases, delivery may occur at the normal time. If the disease is severe, the fetus may require a transfusion while still in your uterus and is usually delivered a few weeks before your due date. This transfusion is performed under ultrasound guidance. The needle is placed through your abdomen and uterus into the abdomen of the fetus. Some babies may require an exchange transfusion after birth if they are born very anemic. Rh negative blood will be given which will not be affected by maternal Rh antibodies still circulating in the fetus's bloodstream.

Q *If I have Rh negative blood and I am going to have a postpartum sterilization, do I still have to receive the Rh immune globulin vaccine?*

A Yes. You may decide to have your sterilization reversed, the procedure may fail to prevent another pregnancy, or, if you need a blood transfusion in the future, the presence of Rh antibodies interferes with crossmatching your blood.

ECTOPIC PREGNANCY

Q *What is an ectopic pregnancy?*

A An ectopic pregnancy is a pregnancy that grows outside of your uterus. The most common site for an ectopic pregnancy is in the fallopian tube (tubal pregnancy).

Q *How common are ectopic pregnancies?*

A Ectopic pregnancies occur once in every 150 to 200 pregnancies.

Q Who is at risk for having an ectopic pregnancy?

A Anyone who has a process that causes partial blockage of the fertilized egg's passage down the fallopian tube. A past history of a tubal infection with gonorrhea or chlamydia increases one's risk, as does past surgery on the tube to correct an infertility problem. Women who become pregnant after a tubal sterilization procedure, on the mini-pill, or with an IUD are at increased risk.

Q What are the symptoms of an ectopic pregnancy?

A Most women miss their menstrual period, and then complain of vaginal bleeding or spotting about 2 weeks later. About half also complain of pain in their lower abdomen, usually on one side. About 1 in 5 women have shoulder pain as well. Lightheadedness or fainting occur in 33% of the cases. Most of these symptoms occur within 6 to 8 weeks after the last normal menstrual period.

Q How does the doctor diagnose an ectopic pregnancy?

A The findings of a positive pregnancy test along with the above symptoms, a uterus smaller than expected for your stage of pregnancy, and a mass on the side of the pain will strongly suggest an ectopic pregnancy. An ultrasound exam may aid in the diagnosis. If the diagnosis is still not certain, a laparoscopy will be performed.

Q Why is an ectopic pregnancy dangerous?

A The pregnancy will expand the tube and then rupture it, causing internal bleeding. If the diagnosis is delayed, massive blood loss, shock, or death may result.

Q What is the treatment for an ectopic pregnancy?

A Removal of the pregnancy must be done. A pregnancy in the tube will never grow for 40 weeks. If future pregnancies are desired and the tube has not ruptured, it may be possible for the doctor to open the tube, remove the pregnancy, and repair the tube. If the tube has already ruptured or future childbearing is not desired, the tube will be removed. At the present time, this surgery is performed through an abdominal incision although in some teaching hospitals it is being performed with the use of laparoscopy (a minor operation usually performed on an outpatient basis under general anesthesia) in selected cases.

Q If I have had an ectopic pregnancy, what are my chances of having another one?

A A repeat ectopic pregnancy may occur in 10% to 20% of subsequent pregnancies.

Q What is my chance of conceiving after an ectopic pregnancy?

A About 50% of women will be able to have a full-term pregnancy after a previous ectopic pregnancy.

PREMATURE RUPTURE OF MEMBRANES

Q What is premature rupture of membranes (PROM)?

A This is a spontaneous break in the amniotic sac before the beginning of labor. There will be leakage of amniotic fluid from your vagina. The initial amount of fluid may be a cup or more or just a few drops of clear, yellow, or greenish fluid. If your water has broken, you will know, because the leaking is continuous or recurrent.

Q What should I do if my membranes rupture?

A Call your doctor. You will be asked to go to the hospital. If you are near term, there are usually no problems. Labor begins in 24 hours in up to 90% of patients. The problem occurs when the membranes rupture prematurely. This may occur in about 10% of pregnancies and is the cause of premature birth in 30% of cases. If PROM occurs between 28 and 34 weeks of pregnancy, about 50% of women will go into labor within 48 hours and 90% will be in labor after 1 week. After a few days in the hospital, the doctor may prescribe bedrest at home, and no baths or sexual intercourse. You will be asked to take your temperature every 4 to 6 hours and report any temperature elevation or abdominal pain, which may indicate an infection of the amniotic fluid. If there are signs of an infection, labor will be induced.

INTRAUTERINE GROWTH RETARDATION

Q How can I tell if my pregnancy is growing normally?

A Many patients ask this question, because a friend or acquaintance will comment that they look smaller or larger than their duration of pregnancy. Doctors screen for abnormal growth of the fetus during each prenatal visit by measuring the fundal height (from pubic bone to top of the uterus).

Q What is intrauterine growth retardation (IUGR)?

A IUGR is a condition that causes a slowing down or cessation of growth of the fetus. When the baby is born, his or her weight will be in the lower 10% for babies of his or her age.

Q Is IUGR dangerous to my baby?

A If the growth retardation is not severe, there is not much danger. But as the weight decreases below the 10th percentile, the risk of stillbirth increases.

Q How common is IUGR?

A It may affect up to 8% of pregnancies in the general population.

Q What are the causes of IUGR?

A
- Small mothers have smaller babies
- Poor maternal weight gain
- Hypertension
- Toxemia
- Women living at very high altitudes
- Severe maternal anemia
- Smoking
- Heroin use
- Cocaine use

- Alcohol abuse
- Twins
- History of a previous growth-retarded infant
- Chronic fetal infections—rubella, cytomegalovirus
- Postterm pregnancy—20% of babies
- Congenital anomalies

Q How does the doctor confirm the diagnosis of IUGR?

A Serial ultrasounds are performed at 2- to 4-week intervals. The doctor will measure the growth of the head, abdomen, and femur and will check for an adequate amount of amniotic fluid to confirm the diagnosis.

Q If my fetus has IUGR and I am close to term, what will happen?

A IUGR stresses the fetus and probably speeds up lung maturity. Since the fetus is in an unfavorable environment, your doctor will elect to deliver your baby. Either induction of labor, if your cervix is ripe and the fetus responded well during a nipple stimulation test, or cesarean section will be performed.

Q What will happen if I am far from term with IUGR?

A If a known cause can be reversed (cessation of smoking, drinking, or drug use), complete bedrest and monitoring of fetal well-being (nonstress test, nipple stimulation test, or biophysical profile) may be employed to gain days or weeks of intrauterine life. If the growth retardation is severe, however, delivery early in the third trimester may be anticipated.

Q What are the possible complications of IUGR?

A Your baby may have to be delivered prematurely, with the possible complication of respiratory distress syndrome of the newborn because of immature lungs. If the fetus undergoes distress during labor, you would require a cesarean section. The presence of meconium and meconium aspiration may occur. There is also an increased incidence of stillbirths.

Q *Are there any problems with these babies later in life?*

A In most cases of IUGR, there is no long-term neurological or intellectual compromise.

PRETERM LABOR

Q *What is preterm labor?*

A Preterm labor is labor that occurs before the 37th week of pregnancy.

Q *How common is preterm labor?*

A Up to 10% of pregnancies end prematurely. Fortunately, only 2% of pregnancies end before 30 weeks—the age before which fetal survival is less than 20%.

Q *What are the causes of preterm labor?*

A The cause in 50% of the cases is unknown. The second most common cause is premature rupture of membranes from unknown causes. Other known causes include: twins, incompetent cervix, congenital anomalies of the fetus, congenital anomalies of the uterus, smoking, poor nutrition, no prenatal care, previous preterm birth, and serious maternal diseases.

Q *How do I know if I am in preterm labor?*

A Many times you don't know. The difference between false labor and real labor is often difficult to establish, so call your doctor if you are unsure.

Q *How does my doctor know if I am in preterm labor?*

A Serial pelvic exams at frequent intervals will show if there is a change in the cervix, establishing the diagnosis of preterm labor. Or, the doctor may place you in the hospital on external fetal monitors, and the display of uterine contractions at least every 10 minutes of at least 30 seconds duration establishes the diagnosis.

Q *Can preterm labor be stopped?*

A Yes, in many cases it can be. The question of whether to stop labor is sometimes controversial and may depend on the reason for labor and the weight and age of your fetus. Initial therapy consists of complete bedrest and hydration with intravenous fluids. This therapy may be successful in almost 50% of cases of preterm labor. Ritodrine or magnesium sulfate administered through the I.V. will be used next, if needed. Success with these drugs may approach 70%. A major factor for stopping labor is the state of effacement and dilatation of the cervix at the onset of therapy. So if you think you are in preterm labor, don't hesitate to call your doctor.

Q *Are there any effects of ritodrine or magnesium sulfate on my baby?*

A There is no increased incidence of birth or developmental defects from these medications.

POSTTERM PREGNANCY

Q *What is a postterm pregnancy?*

A A postterm pregnancy is one that lasts more than 42 weeks from the first day of the last menstrual period. This definition assumes that the length of the previous menstrual cycles was 28 days.

Q *How common are postterm pregnancies?*

A About 10% of all pregnancies last beyond 42 weeks and 3%, more than 43 weeks.

Q *What causes postterm pregnancies?*

A There are many theories, but we don't know the exact cause.

Q *If my first pregnancy was postterm, will this pregnancy be postterm, too?*

A If your first pregnancy was postterm, you have a 50% chance that your second pregnancy will go to 42 weeks.

Q *What are the effects on my pregnancy if it is postterm?*

A Most babies do well even if the pregnancy goes past 42 weeks, but there are potential problems.

In about 20% of these pregnancies, the placenta will not supply enough nutrients to the fetus. Weight loss, decreased amniotic fluid, fetal distress, and meconium aspiration may result.

In another 20% of pregnancies the fetus will continue to grow to at least 9 pounds, 3% of these babies will weigh 10 pounds. These increased birthweights increase the incidence of cesarean section due to cephalopelvic disproportion (the head is too big to make it through the birth canal).

Meconium in the amniotic fluid occurs more commonly, from 27% to 43%. At 40 weeks, the incidence of meconium-stained fluid is about 15%. Meconium may be a warning sign that the pregnancy is being compromised, especially if it is thick and there is little amniotic fluid. Careful internal fetal monitoring during labor will recognize any potential signs of fetal distress.

Q *What will my doctor do if my pregnancy is postterm?*

A Your doctor will monitor the health of your fetus by using nonstress tests, nipple stimulation tests, and/or ultrasound.

If your pregnancy date is accurate and your cervix is ripe, induction of labor will be performed.

If there is a concern for the health of your baby, delivery by induction of labor or cesarean section will be performed.

TWINS

Q *How common are twin pregnancies?*

A In the United States, twin pregnancies occur once in every 93 deliveries. There are two types of twins: identical and fraternal twins. Identical twins come from one fertilized egg that splits early in the pregnancy. Fraternal twins come from two separate fertilized eggs. Fraternal twins are more common, comprising about 70% of twins born.

Q *Are some women more likely to have twins?*

A Fraternal twins are more common if you are a twin or your mother was a twin. Your husband's family history has no influence on the incidence of twins. Twins are also more common with the increasing age and number of pregnancies of the mother. Twins are more common in blacks (1 in 79). Twins are more common with the use of fertility drugs such as Pergonol or Clomid. Identical twins seem not to be influenced by any factors and are constant throughout the world with a birthrate of 1 in 250 births.

Q *How does the doctor know if I have twins?*

A There are some clues that the doctor recognizes. The rapid growth of the uterus after the first trimester, the presence of two heads or buttocks on exam for fetal position, and a large weight gain between visits may indicate the presence of twins. The diagnosis will be confirmed by an ultrasound exam, which is accurate 97% of the time.

Q *Are there any special instructions I should follow if I am having twins?*

A Yes. Having twins is considered a high-risk pregnancy. Twin pregnancies on the average only last up to 37 weeks; there is a greater chance of prematurity. After 28 weeks, many doctors advise their patients to stop working and remain at home, resting for most of the day. Proper nutrition is even more important with a twin pregnancy. Weight gain should be increased to 40 pounds, and iron supplementation is a definite requirement.

Q *Besides prematurity, are there any other potential problems facing me and my babies?*

A Major and minor malformations are twice as common, being 2% and 4%, respectively. There is also a greater chance of morbidity and death of one baby during delivery, the rate being three times as common. Toxemia and placenta previa are more common.

Q *How will I deliver my twins?*

A This will depend on the presentation of the twins at the time of labor and the philosophy of your doctor. In more than 50% of the cases, a vaginal delivery may be expected.

9 Medical Complications of Pregnancy

AIDS

Q *What is AIDS?*

A AIDS stands for Acquired Immune Deficiency Syndrome. AIDS is caused by the AIDS virus, which is also known as Human Immunodeficiency Virus (HIV). This virus attacks the body's lymphocytes (a type of white blood cell), producing immune deficiency. Without this cell-mediated immunity, the AIDS immunocompromised patient is susceptible to unusual infections and cancers. The virus also attacks the nervous system, causing a variety of neurologic and psychiatric conditions.

Q *How common is AIDS?*

A As of March 1987, 33,482 cases of AIDS have been reported to the Centers for Disease Control (CDC) in the United States. Only 2,464 cases of AIDS have been reported in women, the majority of whom were intravenous drug abusers or recipients of infected blood or blood products.

Q *Can you become infected with the AIDS virus and not develop the disease?*

A At the present time, AIDS is a relatively new disease and the actual proportion of infected individuals who may ultimately develop this illness is not known for sure. Right now, it is estimated that about 50% of infected individuals will develop AIDS or AIDS-related conditions (ARC). All infected persons, however, may transmit the virus to others.

Q *How is the AIDS virus transmitted?*

A At the present time, there are four known modes of transmission of the virus: First, through sexual contact with an infected partner; second, by receiving infected blood products; third, by being born to an infected mother; and fourth, by breast-feeding on infected milk.

Q *Should I be tested for the AIDS virus?*

A The following groups of women should be tested for the AIDS virus:
- Women who have evidence of AIDS virus infection
- Intravenous drug abusers
- Women born in countries where heterosexual transmission of the AIDS virus plays a major role
- Prostitutes
- Women whose past or present sexual partners are or were intravenous drug abusers, bisexual, hemophiliacs, or those born in countries where heterosexual transmission is thought to play a major role, or men who have evidence of AIDS virus infection

Since at this time, the prevalence of the AIDS virus in women is so low (0.01%), routine testing of all pregnant women has not been recommended.

Q *If I have been infected with the AIDS virus and I am pregnant, how can I transmit the virus to my fetus?*

A Transmission of the virus takes place during pregnancy, labor, or delivery. One baby was infected by the AIDS virus and was delivered by cesarean section.

Q *What is the risk of transmitting the virus to my fetus?*

A The risk of transmitting the AIDS virus from an infected mother to the fetus is anywhere from 0 to 65%, according to the various studies published to date. We do not know why some women transmit the AIDS virus to their fetus and others don't.

Q *If I have the AIDS virus during my pregnancy and my baby is born without becoming infected, what precautions should I take to prevent him or her from becoming infected?*

A Don't breast-feed. Breast milk has been found to contain the AIDS virus, and one case of transmission of the virus to an infant has implicated breast-feeding.

Q *If I need a blood transfusion, what are my chances of becoming infected with the AIDS virus?*

A Now that all blood donors are screened for the AIDS virus, your risk of contracting AIDS from a blood transfusion is extremely low—only 0.0005%.

HERPES

Q *What is genital herpes?*

A Genital herpes is a viral infection caused by the herpes simplex virus. There are two types, but type II most commonly causes the genital herpes infection. The disease is sexually transmitted. It is extrememly rare to acquire the disease any other way. A flulike illness along with blisters on the vagina, vulva, perineum, buttocks, or thighs occurs with the first outbreak. The blisters will heal in 2 to 4 weeks. Thereafter, the outbreaks occur without fever, and there are usually less blisters formed which heal within 2 weeks.

Q *How common is genital herpes?*

A The incidence is not known for sure, but it has been estimated that 10% to 30% of the population has been infected or exposed. Each year, almost 500,000 new cases occur.

Q *How common is genital herpes in pregnancy?*

A Almost 5% of pregnant women have genital herpes.

Q *If my sexual partner has genital herpes and he has an active lesion, what are my chances of becoming infected?*

A The risk of infection after coming into sexual contact with an infected partner is 60% to 80%. Following exposure to the virus, symptoms such as burning or itching or the appearance of blisters will occur within 1 week.

Q *What are the dangers of a primary genital herpes infection during pregnancy?*

A If the infection occurs in the first trimester of pregnancy there may be a slightly increased risk of miscarriage. Primary infection in the late second or in the third trimester has been associated with preterm delivery.

Q *Is there any treatment for recurrent genital herpes infection during pregnancy?*

A Treatment at this time is symptomatic. Try sitz baths three to four times a day with a betadine solution and ask your doctor for a pain reliever, if needed. Although there is a drug (acyclovir) that is used to prevent recurrent infections and minimize the duration and symptoms of an outbreak, it is not recommended for use during pregnancy at this time.

Q *What is the danger to my baby if I have a genital herpes infection when I go into labor and have a vaginal delivery?*

A If you have a vaginal or cervical infection during labor and have a normal vaginal delivery, up to 50% of babies will become infected. The appearance of blisters will occur by the second week of life. Over half of these babies will die and another one-quarter will have neurological damage.

Q *What will my doctor do if I have a history of genital herpes?*

A First, it is very important to tell your doctor that you or your partner has a history of genital herpes. During the last month of pregnancy, your doctor will perform weekly vaginal cultures for herpes, whether you have an outbreak or not. If you have an active lesion or a positive culture at term, you will have a cesarean section to prevent infection of your baby. If you go into labor with an active infection and you have not ruptured your membranes or the membranes have been ruptured for less than 6 hours, a cesarean section will be performed to prevent infection of your baby. Fortunately, the occurrence of infection at term is rare.

Q *If I have an active herpes infection and a cesarean section, what will happen after delivery?*

A You and your baby will be isolated during your hospital stay. Proper hygiene is recommended, including handwashing and wearing of gloves when you hold your baby. You may breast-feed, if you so desire.

VAGINAL INFECTIONS

Q *What is a trichomonal infection?*

A A trichomonad is a one-celled parasitic organism found in the vaginas of up to 15% of women without symptoms. The infection is sexually transmitted. It is also possible to acquire this infection from communal bathing or sharing wet towels or bathing suits. When infection occurs, you will experience vaginal itching, swelling, and a copious, foul-smelling greenish or grey discharge.

Q *What is the treatment for trichomoniasis during pregnancy?*

A Medications should be avoided during pregnancy if possible. Try douching with vinegar first; this may temporarily relieve your symptoms. If this fails, the use of an antifungal cream or metronidazole (Flagyl, Protostat) may be advised by your physician.

Q *Is a trichomonal infection dangerous during pregnancy?*

A No, this infection does not cause any maternal or fetal complications.

Q *Are yeast infections common during pregnancy?*

A Up to 20% of pregnant women will develop a vaginal yeast infection, usually near the end of pregnancy. Yeast infections are caused by Candida albicans, and pregnancy is the most common predisposing factor for this infection. The symptoms are intense vaginal itching, with swelling and an odorless white creamy or cottage cheese-like discharge.

Q *What is the treatment of a yeast infection during pregnancy?*

A The same treatment applies whether you are pregnant or not. Preparations such as Monistat, Femstat, Gyne-lotrimin, or Mycelex-G all offer effective treatment. You may have to use the medication for a longer period of time; however, these medications are safe during pregnancy.

Q *What are the dangers of a yeast infection during pregnancy?*

A Babies born to women with yeast infections may develop thrush (oral candida infection), a vaginal yeast infection, or diaper rash.

Q *What is a Gardnerella vaginalis (G.V.) vaginitis?*

A This is the nonspecific or bacterial vaginal infection. This infection produces a grey white discharge that is foul smelling and, in a less acidic environment, may smell fishy. The fishy smell may become apparent after intercourse due to the presence of semen.

Q *How is G.V. vaginitis treated during pregnancy?*

A Symptomatic women are treated with metronidazole, ampicillin, or a cephalosporin.

Q *Does G.V. vaginitis cause any complications during pregnancy?*

A No complications have been reported.

Q What is a venereal wart infection?

A Venereal warts, or condyloma acuminata, are caused by the human papilloma virus. They are acquired by sexual contact. These warts may grow on the vagina, vulva, perineum, anus, urethra, bladder, or cervix. Sometimes these warts grow and spread during pregnancy.

Q How is a condyloma acuminata infection treated during pregnancy?

A For the usual small warts, treatment can be by cryosurgery (freezing) or electracautery (burning). These procedures are performed in your doctor's office.

Q What are the complications of a venereal wart infection during pregnancy?

A Although rare, these warts can grow to the size of golf or tennis balls during pregnancy. They are filled with many blood vessels and may cause a massive blood loss. If there is extensive disease and delivery was accomplished by the vaginal route, there have been reports of warts growing near or on the vocal chords of the infants. Most commonly, though, these warts are small, few in number, and do not cause complications.

Q What is a chlamydial infection?

A This is a sexually transmitted disease caused by a bacteria called chlamydia trachomatis. It may infect the cervix or cause a salpingitis (inflammation of the tube). During pregnancy, only the cervix is infected, causing a yellowish discharge, which may be scant and often goes unnoticed.

Q How common is a chlamydial infection in pregnant women?

A The rate of chlamydial infection in pregnancy may be as high as 10%. The most likely women to contract this disease are young, married, pregnant for the first time, and on welfare.

Q *Can a chlamydial infection cause complications during pregnancy?*

A Yes, these pregnancies are more often complicated by premature deliveries, low birthweight infants, and stillbirths or death soon after birth.

Q *Can a chlamydial infection cause problems for my baby after delivery?*

A Yes, up to 60% of babies will contract this infection after a vaginal delivery. A lesser percentage will become infected if a cesarean section was performed after ruptured membranes. Half of these infants may develop conjunctivitis, if not treated with preventative erythromycin ointment, and 10% of babies may develop pneumonia, usually 6 weeks after delivery. There may also be an increased risk of ear and gastrointestinal infections in these babies.

Q *What is the treatment for chlamydial infections during pregnancy?*

A Often, the treatment must start with you alerting your doctor, who would not routinely do a chlamydia culture. The infection is easily treated with a course of erythromycin, which has not been shown to be harmful to your baby.

DIABETES

Q *What is diabetes mellitus?*

A Diabetes is a disease that causes too much sugar to circulate in the bloodstream. The sugar is called glucose.

Q *What is gestational diabetes?*

A Gestational diabetes is diabetes of pregnancy. Hormones from the placenta cause more glucose to appear in the blood. If your body cannot make enough insulin to drive the glucose into your cells for energy, there will be an increase in your blood glucose level.

Q *Which women are more likely to get gestational diabetes?*

A You may have an increased risk of acquiring gestational diabetes if you have one of the following conditions:
- Obesity
- Previous baby weighing at least nine pounds
- Previous stillborn
- Family history of diabetes

However, not all of these women will develop gestational diabetes. Some women who don't have any of these risk factors may develop gestational diabetes. Therefore, all pregnant women are screened.

Q *If I develop gestational diabetes, do I have to take insulin?*

A No, your blood sugar level can be controlled by a diet prescribed by your doctor.

Q *Do gestational diabetics ever develop insulin-requiring diabetes during pregnancy?*

A About 10% of gestational diabetics will develop insulin-requiring diabetes. Therefore, your doctor will take a fasting blood sugar level during each prenatal visit to test for this conversion.

Q *What problems may occur in a pregnancy complicated by gestational diabetes?*

A There is a higher incidence of bladder infections, toxemia, and macrosomia. Macrosomia is a baby that weighs more than 9 pounds. A macrosomic infant has an increased chance of being delivered by a cesarean section. By following the diet and exercise program your doctor prescribes, you will be able to deliver a healthy infant.

MITRAL VALVE PROLAPSE (MVP)

Q *What is mitral valve prolapse?*

A MVP is a minor abnormality of the mitral valve in your

heart. The valve is usually very large and has abundant tissue.

Q *How common is MVP?*

A At least 6% of women have MVP.

Q *What are the symptoms of MVP?*

A Usually you will have no symptoms, but if you do, the most common symptoms are palpitations and chest pain. Other complaints may include: shortness of breath, fatigue, and anxiety—also common complaints of pregnancy.

Q *How will MVP affect my pregnancy?*

A Most women do fine during their pregnancy, without any complications.

Q *Is there an increased chance of my baby having a congenital anomaly if I have MVP?*

A No increased incidence of congenital anomalies occurs in babies of women with MVP.

Q *Will my doctor take any special precautions during my labor?*

A This is a controversial issue; some doctors may give you prophylactic antibiotics during labor.

COMMON VIRAL INFECTIONS

Q *What can I take if I have a cold?*

A If your symptoms are very mild, try drinking large amounts of fluid. This will thin out the mucus in your nose or lungs and relieve the "stuffy" feeling. A vaporizer or humidifier may also help. When you sleep at night, prop yourself up on a few pillows to drain the mucus from your nose and to enable you to breath easier. Sore throats may be soothed by drinking herbal tea with honey. Before you plan on taking any medication during pregnancy, contact your doctor.

Q *Will a cold harm my baby?*

A No. There is no evidence that the common cold causes any birth defects or harms your baby.

Q *What should I do if I have a fever?*

A You should notify your doctor if you have a temperature above 100.4°F. If you have a high fever and flu symptoms, take acetaminophen (Tylenol, Datril, Panadol) to lower your temperature, drink plenty of fluids to replenish what you have lost in perspiration, and stay in bed and rest.

Q *What are the dangers of an influenza viral infection during pregnancy?*

A The complications are essentially the same whether you are pregnant or not. There is no evidence that influenza causes miscarriage or premature labor. Influenza does not cause birth defects.

CYTOMEGALOVIRUS

Q *What is a cytomegalovirus (CMV) infection?*

A CMV is a viral infection. At least 95% of the time the infection is asymptomatic. The remaining 5% have a mononucleosis-like illness (fever, fatigue, sore throat, muscle pain, and lymph node enlargement) that may last from 1 week to 2 months. CMV infection is very common; about 50% of pregnant women in middle to upper socioeconomic groups show evidence of past infection.

Q *How common is congenital CMV infection?*

A Congenital CMV is the most common infection of the fetus. About 1% of infants are born each year with congenital CMV. That's about 30,000 babies per year.

Q *What are the effects of a congenital CMV infection?*

A Severe disease will occur in only 2% to 4% of infected infants, or up to 8,000 per year. These babies may have hearing loss, visual problems, mental or motor retardation, or behavior problems. The disease is fatal in a minority of those infants infected.

Q How do I know if I have developed a CMV infection during pregnancy?

A As I mentioned above, you may not know that you have the infection, and most pregnant women will have been infected before pregnancy.

RUBELLA (GERMAN MEASLES)

Q If my blood tests showed that I was immune to German measles (rubella), should I worry if I am exposed to a child with this disease?

A No. If you are immune, you have already had rubella and you have antibodies in your blood to prevent another infection. At least 85% of women are immune by age 20, and almost 100% by age 35. Many states require a blood test for rubella before obtaining a marriage certificate, and if you are not immune, your doctor will advise you to get the vaccine.

Q If I was not immune to rubella and was exposed to the disease, what will happen to my baby?

A Congenital rubella infection is most devastating when the pregnant woman contracts the disease in the first trimester; up to 50% of the infants may become infected. Later on in pregnancy only about 15% of infants will show evidence of infection. These babies may have cataracts, deafness, or mental retardation. Luckily, since mass vaccination of children began over 20 years ago, congenital rubella has become very rare.

CHICKEN POX

Q If I had chicken pox as a child, should I worry if I come into contact with an individual who has chicken pox?

A No. If you had chicken pox, you cannot contract this viral disease again.

Q If I have never had chicken pox and am exposed, what effects will it have on me and my fetus?

A The risk of congenital malformations due to chicken pox is very rare, even if you contract this disease in your first trimester. Chicken pox infection at term may be complicated by pneumonia.

URINARY TRACT INFECTIONS (UTI)

Q Are urinary tract infections common in pregnancy?

A Infection of the bladder and/or kidney(s) is the most common infection during pregnancy. A UTI may occur in up to 3% of pregnancies in middle- or upper-class women and in up to 10% of those in lower economic classes. The infection may or may not produce symptoms. This is one of the reasons why it is important to bring your urine specimen with you at each prenatal visit; the urine will be examined for evidence of infection.

Q How will I know if I have a bladder infection (cystitis)?

A You may experience one or all of these symptoms: an increased frequency of urination (perhaps every 10 minutes), an increased urge to urinate, pain in your abdomen just above your pubic bone, difficulty beginning to urinate or burning with urination. If you have any of these symptoms, tell your doctor, who will then examine your urine more closely. Remember, you may have these symptoms as a normal result of being pregnant (see page 13).

Q How is cystitis treated?

A There are several different antibiotics that may be safely used during pregnancy. In addition, be sure to drink at least 8 glasses of fluid a day to help flush the bacteria out of your bladder.

Q Will a bladder infection harm my pregnancy?

A The only potential danger is that you may develop a kidney infection, if you are not treated.

Q *How will I know if I have a kidney infection (pyelo-nephritis)?*

A Fortunately, kidney infections are less common than bladder infections, but they are the most common, serious infection that occurs during pregnancy. When they do occur, they are more common on the right side. The most common symptoms are flank pain, fever of 101°F or higher, chills, nausea and vomiting, and/or symptoms of cystitis.

Q *How is pyelonephritis treated?*

A Treatment is best initiated by hospitalization. You will receive an I.V. for two reasons: First, you may be very dehydrated from high fever and excessive perspiration and vomiting. Second, antibiotic treatment through an I.V. is the treatment of choice. With this treatment, 90% of patients will feel better within 2 days.

Q *Is a kidney infection harmful to my pregnancy?*

A If left untreated, a pyelonephritis may possibly cause premature labor.

SURGERY DURING PREGNANCY

Q *Can surgery be safely performed during pregnancy?*

A Yes. Although the need for surgery does not arise too often, if surgery must be performed, you and your fetus will in most instances not be adversely affected.

Q *What are the most common reasons for surgery during pregnancy?*

A The most common operations are for emergency situations: appendicitis, ovarian cysts, gallbladder disease, broken bones, or dental emergencies.

Q *How common is appendicitis during pregnancy?*

A Appendicitis occurs in about 1 in 2,000 pregnancies.

Q *What are the symptoms of appendicitis?*

A You may have nausea and vomiting, right-sided lower abdominal pain, loss of appetite, constipation, and fever. If you have these complaints, report them to your doctor immediately. If an appendectomy is performed, there may be a slight risk of miscarriage or premature labor (depending on your stage of pregnancy), but delay in notifying your doctor and in receiving treatment are more likely to result in these complications and others (ruptured appendix, peritonitis).

Q *What are the symptoms of an ovarian cyst?*

A Most of the time you will be unaware that you have an ovarian cyst. Your doctor may discover a cyst during the pelvic exam on your first prenatal visit.

Q *What is the treatment for an ovarian cyst?*

A Initially, your doctor will wait and observe the growth or disappearance of the cyst. The majority of these cysts may occur normally at the beginning of pregnancy and will spontaneously disappear by the beginning of the second trimester. If not, surgery is usually performed safely around the 16th week of your pregnancy.

Q *Should I have elective surgery during pregnancy?*

A Although such surgery is safe during pregnancy, I do not advise elective surgery, such as cosmetic surgery, be performed during this time.

10 Labor and Delivery

Q *What should I take to the hospital?*

A This is something that you should think about and prepare weeks before your due date and not rush to do right before going to the hospital, especially when you are in labor. You should pack two separate bags: one for labor and one for your postpartum stay.

Your labor bag may contain:
- Chapstick to moisten your lips
- Prepared childbirth cheat-sheet
- A book to read (if you are in early labor)
- Cards or a board game (if you are in early labor)
- Lollipops to keep your mouth moist
- A camera, extra film, and extra batteries
- A pair of socks
- Address book

Your postpartum bag may contain:
- Nursing bras
- Nightgowns (nursing type)
- Bathrobe
- Slippers
- Toothbrush and toothpaste

- Cosmetics
- Hairdryer
- Announcement cards, stamps, and pen
- Loose-fitting clothes to wear home

Q *What is labor?*

A Labor is the occurrence of regular uterine contractions that bring about a change in the cervix—effacement and dilation allowing the fetus to be delivered.

Q *What is effacement?*

A Effacement, which actually may begin before labor, is the thinning of your cervix. The cervix, when not effaced, is from 1 to 2 inches thick, and when completely effaced, as thin as paper. Effacement is described as a percentage—completely effaced is 100%.

Q *What is dilation?*

A Dilation is the progressive widening of your cervical opening. It is measured in centimeters. A completely dilated cervix is 10 centimeters, wide enough to allow passage of the baby into the birth canal, your vagina. Dilation may begin before labor, too, though most women who have had babies (multiparous) may begin labor already dilated 1 to 3 centimeters.

Q *What is station?*

A This refers to the level of the baby's head in relation to the ischial spines, a bony protuberance located in the pelvis and easily felt by your doctor during the pelvic exam. The head felt at the level of the spines is at 0 station; if above, a minus value is given from −1 to −3, then "floating." A positive value is assigned when the head is below the spines, from +1 to +3, then "crowning."

Q *What is engagement?*

A Engagement or "lightening" refers to the drop of your baby's head into your pelvis. With your first pregnancy, this may occur a few weeks before the onset of labor. When it occurs suddenly, you may notice it. You will be aware of an increased pressure in your pelvis and vagina, increased frequency to urinate, easier breathing with less pressure on your rib cage, and less heartburn. With subsequent pregnancies, engagement usually occurs with the start of labor.

Q *What is "show" or "bloody show" or the "mucous plug"?*

A This is a mucous or blood-tinged mucous discharge from the vagina. The mucous plug, which filled the cervical canal, has dislodged. This may occur within hours or several days before labor begins or only after labor has begun. If you have a bloody or mucous discharge after a pelvic exam from your doctor, this is usually not a bloody show.

Q *What is a ripe cervix?*

A This is a condition in which the cervix is soft, at least 50% effaced, and 2 or more centimeters dilated, and the head is engaged, closely applied to the cervix, and at least a −2 station.

Q *What is crowning?*

A The vagina and perineum are distended and about 1 inch of the baby's head is visible in between contractions.

Q *What is pitocin?*

A Pitocin or "pit" is a synthetic form of oxytocin, a hormone produced by the pituitary gland in your brain. Pitocin is given intravenously, if needed, to stimulate uterine contractions. It causes the muscles in the uterus to contract more frequently and with a greater intensity. The effects of pitocin begin working within minutes and last only a few minutes when given through an I.V., so the strength and frequency of the contractions may be accurately controlled.

Q *What are the possible complications of using pitocin?*

A Pitocin is a very potent medication and is used with an internal pressure monitor and fetal scalp monitor to identify and reverse complications. Rarely, hyperstimulation of the uterus, causing prolonged contractions and/or decreased blood flow to the fetus, may occur. Stopping the infusion of the pitocin reverses these complications within minutes.

Q *What is a birthing bed?*

A The birthing bed is one of the truly great advances for the woman in labor. This bed on first glance appears to be your normal hospital bed with all the modern conveniences: electronic controls to raise the head or foot of the bed and wheels. The added modification is the charm. The mattress at the foot of the bed may be taken off and stirrups may be placed at this end to convert the laboring bed into a delivery bed. The laboring woman, with her baby's head crowning, does not have to move to a gurney, wheelchair, or delivery table at this most exciting and (for moving) awkward time. The bed can be moved into the delivery suite and converted or delivery may be accomplished in your labor room.

Q *What is a birthing chair?*

A The birthing chair is a plastic chair that is used in the delivery room for delivery. The bottom of the chair is designed like an open toilet seat cover. There are stirrups and foot pads to rest your feet on in the seating position, and handles for your hands to aid in the pushing process. The birthing chair may be electronically elevated and tilted so your doctor may help in the delivery of your baby.

Q *What is a prep?*

A The nurse shaves the pubic hair located between the bottom of your vagina to the top of your anus, the area where an episiotomy might be performed and repaired. Ask your doctor if this is a routine order.

Q *Why is an enema ordered?*

A The enema is used to evacuate your rectum and lower intestines. This may come as a relief to some women who have been constipated, sensed a pressure in their pelvis, and do not want to have a bowel movement when they are pushing. Many women have had loose stools or diarrhea before entering the hospital and may not need an enema. Discuss the use of enemas with your doctor.

Q *What is false labor?*

A False labor or Braxton-Hicks contractions are irregular contractions of your uterus. These contractions may occur at any time during your pregnancy, but become more common near term. However, you may never experience them. These false labor pains usually last no more than 30 seconds and are really not painful, but they can be annoying. Some women describe them as mild menstrual cramps, others just are aware that their uterus gets hard and their abdomen feels tight. These contractions may occur every hour for several hours or every few minutes for several hours. They will usually disappear if you lie down on your side or walk around.

Occasionally, first-time pregnant mothers cannot tell the difference between false and real labor. Call your doctor if you are unsure. He or she will reassure you by discussing what you are experiencing or by checking your cervix and monitoring your contractions either at the office or in the hospital. Don't feel embarrassed if this happens more than once; some women must be checked for false labor two or more times near term.

Remember, false labor pains are mild, irregular, last less than 30 seconds, are not accompanied by an increased flow of mucus from your vagina, and usually disappear with a change in your position.

Q *How do I know that I am in labor?*

A The signs of labor are regular contractions lasting 45 to 90 seconds, the appearance of a mucous discharge often mixed with blood (show), and/or leaking of amniotic fluid. The contractions often begin at intervals of 15 to 20 minutes, are mild, and may last only 30 seconds. The contractions may occur at this time interval for several hours, or the interval may shorten to 5 minutes within 1 hour. The former usually occurs with your first pregnancy, the latter with a subsequent pregnancy. It is possible that the contractions may begin at 5 minutes apart, especially if you had a quick labor course with a previous pregnancy.

Q Does the baby move during labor?

A Labor does not quiet down the actions of your fetus. He or she will still kick and roll during your labor.

Q Is it normal to have diarrhea at the beginning of labor?

A Yes. Some of the hormonal changes that occur at the onset of labor may provoke diarrhea in some women.

Q When should I call the doctor?

A Discuss this with your doctor. With first pregnancies, I advise my patients to call me when their contractions are 5 minutes apart, last more than 30 seconds from the beginning of one contraction to the beginning of the next, and have been timed for 1 hour. You should also call if your membranes have ruptured, even if you are not in labor. If you had a previous rapid labor (less than 4 hours), call when contractions are 10 minutes apart for 1 hour; they may be 3 minutes apart the next hour, and you could deliver at home, especially if you live far from the hospital. Do not have anything to eat once labor begins. *Remember, drive safely to the hospital; don't speed or drive through red lights.*

Q What happens when I get to the hospital?

A Your doctor will call the hospital, so the personnel will be expecting you. Be sure to preregister at the hospital; making financial arrangements and filling out forms while you are in labor, especially in the middle of the night, can be frustrating. You will then be taken by wheelchair to the labor and delivery area.

Q What are the initial procedures in labor and delivery?

A You are greeted by a nurse who will show you to your room. You will be asked to change into a hospital gown and supply a sample of urine. Your urine will be tested for the presence of sugar, protein, and ketones. You will be asked to get into your labor bed. The external monitors will be placed for listening to your baby's heart and monitoring your contractions. The nurse will perform a vaginal exam, record your blood pressure, temperature, and pulse and observe for signs of labor. She will then call your doctor to relay the information she has gathered and to receive instructions.

Q *What may the doctor order?*

A Some standard orders could be: prep, enema, pain medication, as needed, patient may or may not get out of bed, blood tests, I.V., fluids, or special medications (for preexisting conditions).

Q *What does the labor room look like?*

A Labor rooms in most private hospitals have either one or two labor beds to a room. Usually, there is only one woman in each labor room. The rooms are nicely decorated with patterned wallpaper, pictures, nightstands, a telephone, and a television set. There is an intercom, so you may call your nurse. There will be a fetal monitor in the room and a hookup for oxygen, if needed.

Q *When does the doctor come to the hospital?*

A If all is progressing normally, the doctor will be there for the delivery. If you are admitted in the middle of the night and you are in the early stages of labor, your doctor will see you in the morning. If you are admitted from the office, the doctor will see you after office hours. If this is your first pregnancy, the doctor will come to the hospital just before you start pushing; if you've had a previous birth, when you are in the active phase of labor.

Q *What are the stages of labor?*

A There are three stages of labor. In the first stage, divided into a latent phase and active phase, the cervix dilates to 10 centimeters. In the second stage, the baby descends through the birth canal and is delivered. In the third stage, the placenta is expelled.

Q *What happens during the latent phase?*

A This is the beginning of labor. Your contractions change from being irregular and 15 to 20 minutes apart to 5 to 6 minutes apart. During this phase, the cervix begins to dilate and efface. If this is your first pregnancy, your cervix at the start of labor may be undilated and uneffaced. If this is a subsequent pregnancy, you may begin this phase with cervix dilated from 1 to 5 centimeters and almost completely effaced. The average length is 6 to 7 hours for a primiparous (first-time) and 4 to 5 hours for a multiparous patient. The baby will descend from a −2 to a 0 station. Your contractions will last longer and will feel more uncomfortable near the end of this phase. Most women can carry on conversations, read, watch television, or walk. Many women get to the hospital near the end of this phase.

Q How long can the latent phase last?

A An abnormal latent phase may last more than 20 hours in the primiparous and 14 hours in the multiparous patient.

Q What happens if I have a prolonged latent phase?

A The doctor may give you a sedative or a pain reliever to permit you to sleep. 85% of women will awake in the active phase, 10% will cease contracting (false labor), and 5% may require pitocin.

Q What happens during the active phase?

A Your cervix is 4 to 5 centimeters dilated and 100% effaced. Contractions are now stronger, 45 to 90 seconds long and 2 to 3 minutes apart. You are in the transition stage and appropriate Lamaze or Bradley techniques are being employed. You may not feel like talking now and may become irritable; your sense of humor may be all but lost. The contractions may be quite painful now and you may ask for narcotic medication or an epidural (see page 122). You probably will want to remain in bed and find a comfortable position, although most will change position often during this stage. The baby descends to a +2 station near the end of the first stage. Some women may have the bearing-down sensation or feel like moving their bowels when only 6 to 9 centimeters. If this is your first pregnancy, concentrate on your breathing or relaxation techniques, and, if you feel the need, ask for pain medication to dull this sensation. Pushing against a partially dilated cervix may lengthen this phase by causing swelling of the cervix and partial closing of the opening. Many multiparas (women who have delivered more than one child) may push the cervix from 8 centimeters to complete (10 centimeters) without difficulty and enter the second stage.

Q *How long does the active phase last?*

A From 2 to 4 hours. It may be less than 1 hour in a multipara.

Q *What happens if my active phase is prolonged?*

A You will be stuck at a certain dilation (for example, 6 centimeters) for more than 2 hours. At this point, an I.V. will be started and pitocin will be administered. Usually cervical dilation will resume within 2 hours in 85% of patients, if labor was normal before the arrest of dilation. If progress does not ensue, you will have a cesarean section.

Q *What happens during the second stage of labor?*

A Your baby's head is now in the birth canal at a +2 station. It is time to push your baby out.

Q *How do I know when to push?*

A The pressure of your baby's head causes a reflex, bearing-down sensation. This is involuntary and does not have to be learned. This urge is strongest during a contraction.

Q *How do I push?*

A Wait until you feel the contraction building up and take a slow, deep breath and exhale; then take a deep breath, hold it, and bear down as if you were straining during a bowel movement. Have your coach count slowly to 10, exhale, then inhale rapidly and deeply, hold it, and push to 10 again. You will be able to push 3 times during a contraction. While you are pushing, put your chin on your chest and pull and hold onto your knees. Other positions may be used as long as you are comfortable and pushing effectively.

Q How long is the second stage of labor?

A The average time in primiparas (women giving birth for the first time) is 1 hour, but may be anywhere from 5 minutes to more than 2 hours. The average time in multiparas is 20 minutes, with a range of 1 minute (one push) to 1 hour. The length of time depends on the size of your baby, the size of your pelvis, the position of the baby's head, the quality of your contractions, and the quality of your pushing efforts.

Q What happens if I have a prolonged second stage of labor?

A Your doctor will help deliver your baby by using either forceps or a vacuum extractor, or by cesarean section.

Q What are forceps?

A Forceps are metal instruments that look like salad spoons. They are placed around the top of the baby's head down to the level of his or her ears. Forceps are used to help guide the baby out of the birth canal. At times, the position of the baby's head is not facing straight down and the forceps may help rotate the head and thus provide an easier access for delivery. The vast majority of forceps deliveries occur when the fetal head is stuck after crowning; their use is quite safe. The danger you might have heard associated with forceps delivery occurs when the fetal head is much higher up in the birth canal. Episiotomies are almost always performed with forceps delivery.

Q What are other situations where forceps might be used?

A Besides a prolonged second stage, forceps may be used if the mother's pushing efforts are inadequate, especially after a long labor, the baby's face is not facing down, the head is down in the birth canal and the fetal heart rate displays signs of distress, or (electively) to help deliver women who have epidurals and choose this method.

Q What is a vacuum extractor?

A This is a device that looks like an ice cream cone and is made

of Silastic, a soft, bendable plastic. This device is placed on
the crown of the fetal head and remains attached by applying
variable degrees of suction. The purpose of the vacuum is to
hold station. For example, in a prolonged second stage the
fetal head may come down the birth canal during a contraction only to rise back up into the vagina as the uterus relaxes.
The vacuum will maintain the point of descent of the fetal
head, allowing the next contraction and pushing effort to
advance the fetus down the canal to delivery. The vacuum can
be used in the same situations as the forceps. Ask your doctor
about his or her preference.

Q What happens after the baby's head crowns?

A As the baby descends farther down the birth canal, the
perineum and vagina will distend and thin out. Many women
feel they are being stretched and complain of a burning
sensation. If this is your first pregnancy, you will now be
prepared for delivery.

Q What preparations are made for delivery?

A You will be taken to the delivery room, and your legs will be
placed in stirrups. The nurse will clean your vagina and
perineum. The doctor, now gowned and gloved, will place
sterile sheets over your abdomen and legs. A mirror can be
placed so you may see the birth of your baby. If necessary, an
episiotomy will be performed to deliver your baby.

Q What is an episiotomy?

A An episiotomy is an incision of the vagina and perineum (the
area between the bottom of the vagina and the top of the
rectum) and the muscles underlying this area.

Q When is the episiotomy performed?

A The incision is made when about a 2-inch diameter of the
baby's head is seen during a contraction.

Q How is it performed?

A A pair of curved scissors is used to make the incision.

Q Is there much bleeding from the episiotomy?

A The blood loss is minimal when performed at the proper time, as outlined above.

Q Is anesthesia used?

A Yes, three different types may be employed. If an epidural is in place, this will be more than adequate to numb the area. Local anesthesia or a pudendal nerve block could be used with an agent such as lidocaine.

Q What is local anesthesia?

A This is an injection using a thin needle just under the skin that numbs the nerves in that area. A small pinprick and a burning sensation will be felt during administration of the drug.

Q What is a pudendal nerve block?

A The pudendal nerve supplies the area of the perineum. A long needle is placed in the vagina and an injection is given near the ischial spine. The pain from this injection is minimal. Two injections must be given (one on each side) and pain relief occurs in about 5 minutes. Occasionally, one or both sides of the block do not take and local anesthesia will be used.

Q What is the purpose of an episiotomy?

A It permits an easier and quicker delivery and prevents tearing of the vagina, perineum, and vaginal muscles. It is much easier for your doctor to repair a straight surgical incision than a tear that has raggedy edges.

Q Are there other advantages to an episiotomy?

A Although there has been much debate concerning the widespread use of episiotomies, it has been stated that the number of subsequent surgeries for relaxation of the bladder, vagina, and rectum noted later in life has decreased since the advent of the episiotomy.

Q When is the episiotomy repair performed?

A After the placenta is expelled and the uterus contracts, the doctor will check your cervix and vagina for lacerations and repair these, if necessary. The episiotomy site will then be tested for numbness. Additional anesthesia will be supplied as needed before the repair is begun.

Q How long does the repair take?

A It will take about 10 minutes for the doctor to sew up the episiotomy site.

Q Is there really an extra stitch for the husband?

A No. The vagina, perineum, and muscles will be sewn back together. Kegel exercises will restore the muscle tone in your vagina.

Q Is an episiotomy necessary?

A This varies from doctor to doctor and with certain situations. The procedure is routine for some doctors, while others decide at the time of the delivery. Discuss this with your doctor. When forceps or a vacuum extractor is used, an episiotomy is almost always performed.

Q What happens once the baby's head is delivered?

A The doctor will check for any loops of cord wrapped around the baby's neck and uncoil them. A bulb syringe will then be placed in the baby's mouth and nostrils to remove excess mucus and amniotic fluid. Gentle traction will be placed on the baby's head and you will be asked to push. The baby's shoulders will rotate and will be eased out one at a time. The rest of the baby follows quickly. The baby's nose and mouth will be cleared once again.

Q Where does my baby go after it is born?

A I place the baby on the new mother's (now flatter) abdomen. Don't be afraid to touch your baby, or cuddle and hug him or her.

Q *When does the baby start crying?*

A Your baby will start crying within 1 minute after birth. Crying expands your baby's lungs and begins the normal process of breathing. This also shifts the circulation from fetal to newborn.

Q *Who cuts the cord?*

A Ask your doctor about this one. After a normal delivery, many doctors will let your mate (or significant other) clamp and cut the cord. Ask the nurse to take the photographs.

Q *What is the Apgar score?*

A The Apgar score is physical evaluation of the newborn. It is used to rate the condition of your baby's health after undergoing the stress of labor. The Apgar score was devised by Dr. Virginia Apgar, an obstetric anesthesiologist, in 1958. The ratings are given at 1 and 5 minutes. The best score is a 10, but this is rare; usually the highest score given will be a 9—no one is perfect. Most babies have a score of from 7 to 9 at 1 and 5 minutes. A low score at 1 minute (less than 5) indicates a depressed baby who may require some sort of resuscitation. A low score, less than 5 at 5 minutes, may be associated with an increased risk of neurological problems later in life.

Points	0	1	2
1. Heart rate	Absent	Slow (less than 100)	above 100
2. Respiratory effort	Absent	Slow, irregular	Good, crying
3. Muscle tone	Limp extremities	Some flexion or motion	Active
4. Reflex response to tube in nostril	None	Grimace	Cough or sneeze
5. Color	Blue or pale	Body pink	All pink

Q *Who gives the Apgar score?*

A With a normal delivery, the nurse assigns the Apgar score. After a cesarean section, your pediatrician will do the rating.

Q *What else does the nurse do with my baby in the delivery room?*

A She will take footprints of your baby and place them on the birth certificate (along with your fingerprint), place an identification bracelet around the ankle and wrist (and an identical one on your wrist), and give your baby an injection of vitamin K and place an antibiotic ointment in the eyes.

Q Why does my baby need an injection of vitamin K?

A Newborns do not have an adequate supply of vitamin K, which is necessary for blood clotting.

Q Why is antibiotic ointment placed in my baby's eyes?

A An antibiotic (erythromycin or tetracycline) ointment is administered to prevent an eye infection from gonorrhea or chlamydia transmitted from the mother. Silver nitrate was used in the past, but it was irritating to the newborn's eyes. These ointments are not. Most states require by law that medication be used to prevent these infections.

Q When does the placenta come out?

A Most often the placenta spontaneously separates after 5 minutes, but up to 25 minutes is not abnormally long. You may notice a gush of blood (one cup) and another uterine contraction. Your doctor may ask you to push one last time to complete the delivery of the placenta. If you so desire, ask your doctor to show you the placenta.

Q What happens if the placenta does not detach spontaneously?

A This is a rare event. The doctor will have to manually remove the placenta. A hand is placed in the uterus and shears the placenta off the wall of the uterus. This procedure may be painful but is performed in seconds. If your relaxation breathing does not allow you to manage the pain, ask for a pain reliever.

Q Can I breast-feed my baby right after he or she is born?

A As long as everything has progressed normally, you can try. Most babies aren't that hungry right after their trip down the birth canal; they'd rather get warm and breathe. Most babies will start nursing about 20 minutes after birth.

Q *What happens after the placenta is expelled?*

A There is usually some bleeding and clots of blood following the placenta. Your uterus may not contract right away and bleeding may continue. To contract the uterus, you may try nursing your baby—stimulation of your nipple causes the release of oxytocin—the doctor will firmly and gently massage your uterus, causing it to contract, or the nurse will give you an injection of pitocin into a muscle or an I.V. to cause uterine contractions. Discuss which method your doctor employs. It is important for your uterus to contract to prevent excessive blood loss.

After the delivery of the placenta, you may develop some tremors or the "postpartum shakes." This is quite normal. Your body has just been through a great deal of exercise. The shakes only last a couple of minutes.

Your doctor will then examine your cervix and vagina for any possible tears and repair them along with the episiotomy, if one was performed. Your nurse will then clean you up and you will be taken out of the delivery room. Many hospitals allow family members or friends to wait just outside the labor and delivery area and greet the new family just before going to the recovery room.

Q *Can my partner give the baby a bath after birth?*

A Giving your new baby a bath after delivery is part of the Leboyer method of delivery. Dr. Frederick Leboyer, a French obstetrician, has developed a delivery method that he feels will minimize the trauma of birth. He recommends dim lighting, a quiet atmosphere, placing the baby on the abdomen after birth, clamping the cord after its pulsations have stopped and a warm bath to acclimatize the newborn to its new environment.

Q *What happens in the recovery room?*

A You will stay in the recovery room for about 1 hour. During this time, the nurses will check your blood pressure, pulse, and temperature every 15 minutes. In addition, your fundus will be massaged to assure it has contracted and you will be examined for the quantity of blood flow. In most hospitals, your husband and baby may accompany you and stay with you in the recovery room. If you are hungry, food will be served.

ANALGESICS AND ANESTHESIA
FOR LABOR AND DELIVERY

Q If I need relief from the pain of labor, what is available?

A Sedatives, narcotics, tranquilizers, epidural, or spinal anesthesia may be given to provide pain relief during labor. You must ask for something for pain relief if you want it.

Q When would my doctor give me a sedative?

A Sedatives such as Seconol are given in the latent phase of labor if you cannot rest when the contractions are still irregular. The sedative may be given as a pill or an intramuscular injection.

Q What are the effects on me?

A The sedative should make you drowsy and allow you to sleep until the contractions become more regular and forceful. If you are in labor, a sedative will not slow it down.

Q What are the effects on the fetus?

A The same as on you, drowsiness and sleep. Sedatives are usually only given, if needed, in the latent phase of first pregnancies, so the effects of the drug on the fetus have worn off long before delivery.

Q When are narcotics given?

A Narcotics are given in the late part of the latent phase and during the active phase.

Q How effective are narcotics in relieving pain?

A With moderate pain, relief is attained up to 80% of the time. Narcotics also reduce the anxiety you may experience due to the pain of labor.

Q How are narcotics administered?

A Narcotics are given by either intramuscular injection or through an intravenous line.

Q *Will narcotic medication slow my labor?*

A No! In fact, your labor may be shortened by the medicine.

Q *Which narcotics may be used?*

A Demerol is one of the most common drugs used. Others are Nubaine or Stadol.

Q *How fast does Demerol work and how long do the effects last?*

A If given through your I.V., you will start to feel the effects within 1 minute. Maximal pain relief will occur in 5 minutes and last for about 1 to 2 hours, depending on the dose given. If an intramuscular injection is given, pain relief will begin in about 10 minutes, have maximal effect in 45 minutes, and last from 3 to 4 hours, again depending on the dose administered.

Q *What are the side effects of narcotic medication on me?*

A Drowsiness, nausea and vomiting, and respiratory depression may occur.

Q *Can I have a medicine to prevent these side effects?*

A Yes, as a matter of fact, many doctors give a tranquilizer with the narcotic to prevent the nausea and vomiting. In addition, the tranquilizer (Phenergan, Vistaril) will add to the effects of the narcotic. This means that less of the narcotic will be given to effect the same degree of pain relief.

Q *What are the side effects on the fetus or baby?*

A The narcotic will enter the fetal circulation in 1 to 5 minutes depending on the route of administration. The side effects are the same as above. Your doctor will not administer a narcotic close to delivery to avoid respiratory depression of your baby at birth. If this happens, however, a narcotic antagonist may be given to the baby to reverse the effects.

Q *Are there any long-term effects on my baby?*

A There are no neurological or developmental effects on the baby.

Q *What is an epidural?*

A It is an injection of a local anesthetic through your back and in between the segments of your bony spine into the epidural space, a potential space between the dura (the covering membrane of the spinal cord and fluid) and the surrounding tissues.

Q *Who gives it?*

A It is administered by the anesthesiologist.

Q *How does it work?*

A The nerves leaving and entering the spinal column are bathed in the local anesthetic and are numbed.

Q *What special preparations are needed before placement?*

A You will need an I.V. for hydration and internal monitors to more closely observe the uterine contractions and fetal heart rate. A blood pressure cuff will be placed on your arm to monitor your blood pressure at short intervals after the epidural is activated.

Q *When can I ask for one?*

A As soon as you feel that the pain is unbearable. This usually occurs during transition. Some women who had pain with prior pregnancies will request an epidural in early labor before the pain becomes too intense. An epidural at this time may slow labor considerably, widening the interval between contractions. Pitocin may be used in this situation to enhance labor.

Q *How soon will I have pain relief?*

A Usually in about 20 minutes. First, the anesthesiologist will give you a small test dose of the drug and observe for side effects. If none occur after 10 minutes, a full dose will be given. Its effects will be appreciated in 10 minutes.

Q What will I feel?

A You will feel no more pain from uterine contractions; in fact, you will not even feel them. You will be numb from the top of your uterus to the tips of your toes!

Q How long does the anesthesia last?

A Depending on the type of local anesthetic used, the effects may last from 45 minutes to 2½ hours. In addition, a catheter (tube) may be placed in the epidural space for repeated administration of the anesthetic, as needed.

Q What are the advantages?

A Clearly the main advantage is pain relief. Another plus occurs in the previously agitated mother in intense pain and slow progress in labor—the relief of pain may quicken cervical dilation and relax the muscles of the pelvic floor, hastening the end of the first stage of labor. Also, with the catheter in place the anesthesiologist can selectively provide pain relief to the perineum during the second stage of labor or administer anesthesia for a cesarean section, if one becomes necessary.

Q In what circumstances should an epidural not be placed?

A If there is heavy vaginal bleeding, an infection near the injection site, previous back surgery, or neurological disease.

Q What complications may occur?

A The following complications may occur, though they are rare. The anesthetic may be ineffective. A spinal anesthesia may be inadvertently administered, leading to complications of a spinal. Hypotension (low blood pressure) may be induced. Rarely, convulsions can occur if the local anesthetic is injected into a blood vessel instead of the epidural space. If the first stage of labor ends before the effects of the anesthetic wear off, the mother will not have the bearing-down reflex and may not push effectively enough to deliver her baby, thus lengthening the time spent in the second stage of labor.

Q *What are the effects on the baby?*

A With the properly selected anesthetic agent, there is minimal transfer of drug to the fetus, since the drug is broken down by plasma and placenta.

Q *What is spinal anesthesia?*

A This is anesthesia provided by injecting the anesthetic agent into the spinal cord.

Q *How is it given?*

A The same way as with the epidural, only the needle punctures the dura and the drug bathes and numbs the nerves in the spinal column.

Q *What are the effects of spinal anesthesia?*

A Complete loss of sensation and muscle function in the area the nerves anesthetized supply.

Q *When is it given?*

A Spinal anesthesia is given right before a forceps delivery, if needed. When given for a forceps delivery, it is called a "saddle block," because the area of the body affected is that which would touch a saddle if you were to sit on one. Spinal anesthesia may also be used as anesthesia for a cesarean section; in this case, the area of your body affected would be from your navel down to your toes.

Q *What are the possible complications of a spinal anesthesia?*

A The most notorious complication is a spinal headache, which actually occurs in less than 1% of patients. As with an epidural, low blood pressure and a total spinal anesthesia may rarely occur. Meningitis is an extremely rare complication.

MECONIUM

Q What is meconium?

A Meconium is the dark green feces of the fetus (or newborn). If the fetus has a bowel movement while in your uterus, the fluid may be yellowish, light green, or dark green, depending on the amount of meconium passed and the amount of amniotic fluid present. Similarly, the consistency of the meconium-stained fluid may be watery or like pea soup.

Q Why does the baby pass meconium?

A Your fetus may pass meconium as a response to the compression of his or her umbilical cord or to a decrease in oxygen supply. Or it may be a normal bodily function of the mature fetus.

Q How common is meconium?

A Meconium-stained amniotic fluid may be seen in up to 20% of pregnancies at term and up to 40% at 42 weeks.

Q What is the significance of meconium?

A Meconium by itself does not indicate that your fetus is in distress. But if your fetus does exhibit signs of distress during labor, there is a greater chance of a lower Apgar score at birth. There is also a greater chance that the fetus will do poorly during labor, if there is thick meconium present.

Q What does the doctor do if I have meconium during labor?

A Your doctor will use the internal fetal monitors to more closely monitor the response of your fetus during labor. After the delivery of your baby's head, your doctor will carefully suction out any meconium in your baby's nose and throat and will continue to do so as the body is being delivered. If the meconium is thick, your doctor will cut the umbilical cord and take your baby to the warmer to look at your baby's vocal cords and suction out the trachea for any remaining meconium. This is done to prevent meconium from being aspirated into the baby's lungs, a situation that could cause inflammation of the lungs and breathing problems in the newborn.

Q *What is "back labor"?*

A "Back labor" is so named because the pains of labor are felt most intensely in the back.

Q *Why do some women experience "back labor"?*

A The intensity of labor pains or where the pains are felt the most depends on the individual and her nervous system.

Q *Is labor more common during a full moon?*

A Although both doctors and patients seem to believe that the moon influences the onset of labor, this is not so. This myth was dispelled by Dr. Witter, who demonstrated through an elaborate study that the full moon had no influence on the number of deliveries or on women in active labor (in Baltimore, at least).

Q *Are more babies born in the middle of the night?*

A Fortunately for your doctor and possibly you, no. The percentage of babies born throughout the day is about equal.

INDUCTION OF LABOR

Q *What is induction of labor?*

A The doctor will artificially rupture your membranes (break your water) using an instrument called an amnihook. This procedure is done rapidly and is usually only as uncomfortable as a pelvic exam. The amnihook looks like a crochet needle and it snags and tears the amniotic sac. Oftentimes, if your cervix is ripe, this will initiate the start of uterine contractions within 1 to 2 hours. If labor does not ensue, an I.V. for pitocin induction will be started to initiate and maintain uterine contractions.

Q *What are some medical indications for induction of labor?*

A • Mild PIH (toxemia) at term or severe PIH near term
• Postterm pregnancy

- Rh disease
- IUGR
- Decreased fetal movement with an unreactive NST at term
- Diabetes mellitus at term

Q *What about an elective induction of labor?*

A An induction may be performed when there is a previous history of rapid labor (less than 4 hours) or if false labor is bothersome enough to cause sleeplessness. A particular date close to term might also be chosen, if the cervix is ripe. The choice of this procedure for these reasons, however, should be discussed with your doctor.

Q *What are the advantages?*

A If you have a history of rapid labor, a home or in-transit delivery will be avoided. The induction is usually begun in the morning, and therefore a good night's sleep before labor begins can be expected. The expectant mother will be told to fast overnight so the possibility of vomiting food will be eliminated. There will be a full complement of nurses, operating crew, and anesthesiologists present during a day-time induction, if a problem arises. Prior arrangements can also be made regarding your partner's schedule and care for your other children.

Q *What are the potential complications?*

A If the cervix is ripe, the pregnancy near term, the head engaged and closely applied to the cervix, induction by amniotomy with or without pitocin poses no potential problems. However, if the cervix is not ripe, the induction could be lengthy and unsuccessful, requiring a cesarean section. If the pregnancy is not close to term, the baby can be born with immature lungs, leading to respiratory complications at birth. If the head is not engaged, a prolapsed umbilical cord may result, leading to an emergency cesarean section. The complications of pitocin have been discussed previously (see page 108).

Q *How many hours will my labor last if I am induced?*

A Length of labor depends on the condition of the cervix (dilation and effacement) at the start of the induction and past labor history. For example, if this is your first pregnancy and your cervix is only 1 centimeter dilated and 50% effaced, your first stage of labor could last 12 hours or more. But if this is your third pregnancy, your cervix is dilated to 3 or 4 centimeters, and you are completely effaced, your first stage of labor may be only 1 or 2 hours following onset of regular contractions.

Q *Are the uterine contractions more painful if I have an induction of labor with pitocin?*

A No. Pitocin will cause your uterus to contract just as hard as if you went into labor spontaneously. In fact, although the uterine contractions will initially register strong on the internal monitors, you will not perceive them as such until your cervix completes its effacement and starts to dilate.

11 Cesarean Section

Q *What is a cesarean section (C/S)?*

A A C/S is a major surgical operation performed by your doctor to deliver your baby by an incision made through your abdomen.

Q *What are the indications for a C/S?*

A The most common reasons for a C/S are the following:
- A previous cesarean section, if indicated or desired (see VBAC, on page 136)
- Your cervix fails to dilate completely
- Your pelvis is too small to allow the baby to descend through the birth canal (cephalopelvic disproportion)
- Fetal distress
- An abnormal fetal position (i.e., the feet or back would be delivered first)
- Placenta previa
- Rh disease
- Severe PIH (toxemia) with an "unripe" cervix
- Diabetes with a large fetus
- Prolapse of the umbilical cord through the dilated cervix

- Previous uterine surgery (i.e., removal of a fibroid tumor)
- Pelvic tumor obstructing the birth canal
- Active genital herpes or a positive herpes culture at term

Q Who does the C/S?

A Your doctor performs the surgery with another doctor assisting, either his partner or an associate. Some obstetricians use a family doctor as an assistant.

Q What happens before I have the C/S?

A Your doctor will explain to you the reason for the C/S and the potential complications. You will then sign a consent form for the procedure. Your nurse will then prepare you for the surgery. A Foley catheter will be placed in your bladder to keep it drained; this is done to prevent an injury to the bladder during the surgery. You will need an I.V. for the administration of medications, if needed, during surgery. The pubic hair on your abdomen will be shaved, to clean the area where your doctor will make the incision. Blood will be taken for a CBC, blood type, and Rh titer to crossmatch your blood in case a blood transfusion is necessary. A test will also be performed to see that your blood clots properly. If the C/S is not a life-threatening emergency for you or your fetus, the anesthesiologist will discuss the different types of pain relief that can be used during the operation. All this is done in the labor room. You will then be transported to the operating room, usually located in the labor and delivery room area, and moved onto the operating table. If a spinal or epidural anesthesia was selected, the anesthesiologist will place this now. You will lie on your back and your legs will be strapped down to prevent them from moving during the operation, if general anesthesia is given, or from falling off the table, if a spinal or epidural was given. The anesthesiologist will monitor your blood pressure with a blood pressure cuff and your heart with electrocardiogram leads, which he or she will place on your chest. A nurse will place a pad on your leg to ground you, if the doctor chooses to use cautery for hemostasis during the procedure. Your abdomen will then be washed and sterile drapes will be placed over your body, except for the site of the incision.

Q *Can my partner watch the C/S?*

A Most doctors and hospitals allow the partner to be present during the cesarean section. He is usually asked to sit on a stool right by your head, so that he may hold your hand and talk to you (if you are awake) during the surgery. A drape usually blocks his view of the surgery, but he can if he chooses stand up and watch any part of the C/S. Depending on the hospital, he may even be allowed to take photographs.

Q *Can I watch the C/S?*

A Some operating suites are equipped with mirrors and these can be set up for you to view the surgery, if you so desire.

Q *How is the C/S performed?*

A An incision is made with a scalpel (surgical knife) through the skin of the abdomen. Two types of skin incisions can be done: a vertical incision from the top of the pubic bone to the navel or a horizontal incision about 4 inches long placed two finger-widths above the pubic bone (the so-called bikini cut). The bikini cut is most commonly used in my practice, but ask your doctor which incision he or she uses. The muscles of the abdomen are separated and the peritoneum is entered (the lining of the abdominal contents). The bladder is pushed down away from the uterus and an incision is made in the uterus. Two types of uterine incisions can be made here, horizontal or vertical; the horizontal incision is made more commonly. The fetus is then delivered through this incision, the mouth suctioned, the cord clamped and cut, and he or she is given to the pediatrician. The placenta is delivered next, and then the uterine and abdominal incisions are closed in layers.

Q *How long does a C/S take?*

A The average time is about 45 minutes.

Q *Who is in the delivery room during a C/S?*

A There are quite a few people: you, your mate, your doctor and his or her assistant, the anesthesiologist, your pediatrician, a scrub nurse to hand the instruments to the doctor, a circulating nurse to get extra equipment, if needed, a nursery nurse, a labor room nurse, and finally your new baby!

Q *What are the potential complications of a C/S?*

A Cesarean section has become one of the most common surgical procedures performed in this country. Complications can and do occur, but they are rare. Infection of the uterus, bladder infection, excessive blood loss, and injury to the urinary tract (bladder, ureters, and kidneys) are the most frequent complications. The incidence of uterine and bladder infections has decreased since the use of prophylactic antibiotics. Another rare event is an infection of the skin incision. Death of the mother is a very rare event. Trauma to the baby during delivery is less likely during a C/S delivery than a vaginal delivery. Complications from anesthesia are infrequent and transient.

Q *If I am having an elective primary or repeat cesarean section, can I donate my own blood, or can a family member or friend donate blood for me, in case I need it?*

A Yes. Hospital blood banks now have programs where you or your family or friends may donate blood in advance of your surgical procedure. Programs such as the Autologous Blood Donations or Directed Blood Donations have been implemented because of the fear of acquiring AIDS through a blood transfusion. However, the risk is exceedingly low (0.0005%), since AIDS testing of blood has been instituted. Autologous blood donations must be done within 35 days of the surgery and directed blood donations, within 3 to 5 days of the surgery. Of course, a directed blood donor must have the same blood type and Rh factor as you do.

Q *When can I breast-feed my baby after a C/S?*

A If an epidural or spinal block was used for anesthesia, you will be able to begin breast-feeding in the recovery room, after your vital signs have been taken. If you had general anesthesia, you will be groggy for about an hour after the surgery, but as soon as you are awake you may start breast-feeding your baby.

Q *Will I be in much discomfort after my C/S?*

A Unfortunately, the answer is yes. You have undergone major abdominal surgery and this hurts. Of course, everyone has a different threshold for pain, and so you will hear different impressions from your friends. The pain is most severe the day of surgery. You will require pain medication, and this will be provided by your doctor as needed. The pain is more severe in mothers who were in labor and who then needed a C/S. Repeat or elective primary C/S moms do much better and feel better faster. Injections of pain relief medication, such as Demerol, are given on the day of surgery and the first postoperative day; thereafter, pills for pain relief are more than adequate. By the end of your first postoperative day, however, you are starting to feel much better. By the time you leave the hospital—from 3 to 5 days after the C/S—you will feel the need for medication only occasionally.

Q *What happens to me after the C/S?*

A That night—as with a vaginal delivery—excitement and happiness may cause insomnia. Your diet that day will consist of ice chips and sips of clear liquids. Your I.V. will remain in place from 24 to 48 hours. You will be allowed to shower as soon as the I.V. is removed; you may get your incision wet. The Foley catheter will be removed from your bladder on the morning of your first postoperative day. You will be asked to walk; early ambulation leads to early recovery! A clear liquid or regular diet will be ordered for you on your first postoperative day, although you may not be hungry until later that day or the next day. Your abdomen may become distended with intestinal gas on the second or third postoperative day, and you will look pregnant again. The best way to prevent this is to walk. Most mothers have a bowel movement by the fourth postoperative day. Skin staples, if used, will be removed on the day you leave the hospital.

Q *When can I leave the hospital?*

A The length of your hospital stay depends on how fast your

body recovers. Most patients are ready to go home by the fourth or fifth day after the cesarean section; some patients will be ready to leave on the third postoperative day. Don't rush home, especially if you will have no help at home. Remember, you now have to care for yourself and your new baby.

Q Is there a limit to the number of cesarean sections I can have?

A No. There is really no increased risk of uterine rupture with subsequent pregnancies and cesarean sections.

VAGINAL DELIVERY AFTER CESAREAN (VBAC)

Q I had a cesarean section with my first baby. Do I need to have another cesarean section or can I try to deliver vaginally?

A The rule "once a cesarean, always a cesarean" now does not apply to everyone. If certain criteria are met, you may elect to have a trial of labor. The criteria are:
- The incision on the uterus was in the lower segment and made transversely. The vertical or classical incision has a high probability of rupturing during labor (1%).
- The reason for the previous cesarean section has not occurred in the present pregnancy. For example, placenta previa or breech presentation.
- The fetus weighs under 9 pounds.

Q If my first C/S was for CPD (cephalopelvic disproportion), how good are my chances of delivering vaginally?

A Your chances of having a normal delivery will be between 66% and 77%—very good odds for a second try.

Q If my C/S was for a breech, what are my chances?

A Up to 90% of women will be able to deliver vaginally.

Q *If my C/S was for fetal distress, what are my chances?*

A From 70% to 85% will have a normal delivery.

Q *What are the dangers of a vaginal birth after C/S (VBAC)?*

A In one large study of over 1,200 VBAC deliveries, there were no fetal or maternal deaths. The risk of the low transverse uterine scar rupturing is rare; the scar may separate in almost 3% of cases, but does not cause a problem.

Q *What special procedures are done during labor?*

A Most hospitals have special policies for VBAC, such as:
- The laboring patient will have an I.V.
- Internal monitors will be used during labor.
- The doctor must be in the hospital when the patient is in active labor.
- A consent form for C/S will be signed.
- Preoperative blood work will be drawn.
- Anesthesia coverage will be available for emergency C/S.

12 Postpartum

Q *How should I take care of my episiotomy?*

A Your nurses will show you how to clean your episiotomy site after urinating. You will be supplied with a peri-bottle, which is filled with soap and water and used to douse this area. Remember to always wipe your perineum from front to back and use each piece of toilet paper only once.

Q *What can I use to relieve the pain from the episiotomy?*

A I like to have my patients wear an ice pack for 24 hours after delivery, if they have had an episiotomy. The cold decreases the swelling that normally accompanies an injury (episiotomy in this case) and also numbs this area, providing very good pain relief in most cases.

After the first day, a heat lamp or warm sitz baths for 20 minutes, three times a day, will help to minimize the discomfort. There are also anesthetic creams available to put on the episiotomy; your doctor will probably order one of them as well as mild pain relievers.

Q *Can my stitches break, and will the episiotomy open up?*

A It would be extremely rare for the stitches to break, but if they should, do not worry. The skin edges are closed by a tight seal of serum within 6 hours. In fact, years ago, the skin was closed by clamps that were left on for several hours and then removed!

Q *Do I have to get the episiotomy stitches removed?*

A No. The sutures dissolve in 3 to 6 weeks. You may notice some pieces of suture in your lochia (discharge from your uterus), but don't worry, your vagina has already healed.

Q *How long will I have discomfort from the episiotomy?*

A It may bother you for a week or two, or just a day or two. If the pain lasts longer or becomes worse, call your doctor. Some women have more pain from their hemorrhoids than from the episiotomy.

Q *Can I walk up stairs if I had an episiotomy?*

A Sure, but don't climb stairs two or three steps at a time. If the episiotomy site hurts when you climb stairs, limit the number of times you must use them during the day.

Q *What are "afterpains"?*

A "Afterpains" are uterine contractions that may cause some discomfort after the delivery of your baby. This pain is most noticeable during nursing. Nursing stimulates your pituitary gland to release oxytocin, which, in addition to causing the muscle cells around your milk ducts to contract, will cause your uterus to contract. This will empty your uterus of any residual blood and tissue. The cramping pain is more common with subsequent pregnancies and may last for up to a week. If you are very uncomfortable, ask your doctor for a mild pain reliever.

Q *How long will I bleed postpartum?*

A Whether or not you are breast-feeding, you may bleed for up to 6 weeks. The bleeding is heaviest the first few days after delivery and then may start and stop with bleeding, spotting, or clotting. Or you may bleed for only a week.

Q **What is lochia?**

A Lochia is the discharge from your uterus. The first few days after delivery it is red, due to the bleeding. After a few days, when the bleeding stops, the lochia is pale. After about 2 weeks, the lochia may turn white and have a characteristic and, to some, unpleasant odor. The lochia will disappear within 3 to 6 weeks.

Q **I passed large clots, is that abnormal?**

A Passing clots may occur during the first postpartum week and is normal. The slow discharge of blood from your uterus collects in your vagina and coagulates, forming a clot. Typically, you will pass these clots when you increase your abdominal pressure, which will force the clot out of your vagina. This may occur when you cough, sneeze, get out of bed, or have a bowel movement.

Q **What kind of bleeding is abnormal?**

A A heavy flow of fresh, bright-red blood is abnormal, and you should notify your doctor immediately. This is a rare occurrence. If it does happen, however, it will appear about 2 to 4 weeks after delivery and is due to slow healing of the placental site or retained placental tissue. Treatment with methergine will usually stop the bleeding, although a D&C may sometimes be necessary.

Q **Should I prepare my nipples for breast-feeding?**

A No special preparation is necessary to ready your nipples for breast-feeding. A study has shown that pregnant women who only prepared one nipple, by either rubbing, rolling, massaging with creams, or pulling, reported no difference in sensation between the prepared and unprepared sides.

Q **Can I breast-feed if I have inverted nipples?**

A Sure. If you have inverted nipples, you can use the Hoffman technique to evert them. Starting at about 34 weeks, place your index fingers at the edges of your areola and press it inward and away from your nipple. Move your fingers 90° away and repeat. Do this twice a day.

Q Do I have to feed my newborn infant any other foods if I am breast-feeding?

A Human milk is the most appropriate nutrient for your baby, according to the American Academy of Pediatrics. The American College of Obstetricians and Gynecologists believes that breastmilk alone will provide all the nourishment required for most babies during the first 4 to 6 months of life.

Q What are some other advantages of breast-feeding?

A Breastmilk offers immunologic protection against many types of disease, allergy, and infection. Breast-fed babies are ill less often and are hospitalized less for infection than formula-fed babies. Breast-fed babies are not as likely to become obese. Breast-feeding is economical; you don't have to buy it. It is easy to transport your baby's food around with you. It is convenient—nothing to prepare, nothing to buy. Breast-feeding helps contract your uterus and shrink it back down to its prepregnancy size faster. Breast-feeding also works as a natural contraceptive agent, to some degree.

Q If I have small breasts, will I produce enough milk to properly nourish my baby?

A Yes. The size of your breasts does not matter. Breasts are mostly made up of fat—the larger the breasts, the more fat content. Breastmilk does not come from breast fat. Breastmilk is made from the breast glands, which make up only a small part of the breast. Breast glands enlarge during your pregnancy and after delivery, however.

Q When should I start breast-feeding?

A Start breast-feeding your baby as soon as he or she has warmed up after delivery. If this is your first baby, ask your nurse to show you how.

Q How should the baby suck on my breasts?

A Your baby should suck on as much of the areolar area as he or she can, so that the milk is emptied from the ducts. The strength of the suction is not important; very little force is required to empty the breast reservoirs.

Q How can I prevent sore nipples?

A By having your baby suck on the areola and not just the nipple. Also, insert your finger into the corner of your baby's mouth to break the suction after feeding.

Q How long will it take for my milk to come in?

A The appearance of breastmilk may occur anytime after delivery for up to 10 days. The milk usually appears on the 3rd or 4th day after delivery. In the meantime, your baby will nurse on colostrum.

Q How long should I breast-feed at each feeding?

A At the beginning, limit your feedings to 5 or 6 minutes on each breast then gradually increase to 10 or 12 minutes per breast. The baby gets most of the breastmilk during the first 6 to 7 minutes of the feeding. After a while, you may want to nurse for longer periods of time. Some mothers like to nurse, and some babies like to suckle. If you don't have the additional time, have your baby use a pacifier. You do not have to feed the baby any additional food or water; breastmilk is enough.

Q How often should I breast-feed my baby?

A Most breast-fed babies should be nursed every 3 to 4 hours during the first month. Usually, he or she will let you know that it is time to eat. But if not, you should try to feed your baby at least six times a day.

Q How can I increase my supply of breastmilk?

A First, if you think you do not have enough milk, call your pediatrician and discuss this. If your pediatrician agrees that you should increase your milk stores, then step up your feedings to every 2 hours during the day and at least every 3 hours at night. Also, try to get a little more rest and drink more fluids. After a few days, you will have more milk with each feeding. There is no specific food or beverage that will increase the quantity or quality of your breastmilk.

Q *Can I diet if I am breast-feeding?*

A Unless you are extremely obese, you really shouldn't. The breast-feeding mother requires an additional 500 to 1,000 calories a day. This can be accomplished by drinking a quart of skim milk and eating an egg each day. Since breast-feeding requires calories, you will lose weight more easily and quickly than your non-breast-feeding friends without actively dieting.

Q *Should I avoid certain foods when I am breast-feeding?*

A No, not in the beginning. There are really very few foods that will disturb your baby. After a few weeks, if you suspect that one particular food or spice is upsetting your baby, eliminate it from your diet.

Q *Should I discontinue breast-feeding if I catch a cold or the flu?*

A No, breastmilk will not transmit these viruses to your baby. These infections are transmitted by water droplets from your nose or mouth. The baby will become sick, whether you breast- or bottle-feed, if you are not careful about preventing transmission of your germs.

Q *If I am under stress or have a lot of anxiety, will my milk dry up?*

A No, your emotional state will not interfere with your milk production. However, it may be harder for your milk to come down. If you are having this problem, sit or lie down for a few minutes before you breast-feed and relax.

Q *If I am having problems breast-feeding, whom can I call for help?*

A Call your pediatrician first. If you need additional help, try

La Leche League International. This organization has chapters all around the country. Their address is:

La Leche League International
9616 Minneapolis Ave.
P.O. Box 1209
Franklin Park, IL 60131

They also have a 24-hour hotline: (312) 455-7730.

Q *If I am breast-feeding, do I have to use contraception?*

A Only if you don't want another child right away! Breast-feeding usually does delay the onset of your first ovulation for at least 10 weeks after delivery and can suppress ovulation for much longer periods of time, but it is not the best form of contraception. Also, you may ovulate *before* you have your first menstrual period after delivery, so you can become pregnant without really knowing when it happened. If you are not planning to increase the size of your family right away, talk to your doctor about contraception before you leave the hospital.

Q *What kind of contraception can I use when I am breast-feeding?*

A Foam combined with condoms, an IUD, a diaphragm, the sponge, and the minipill are all effective methods of contraception that can be used while you are breast-feeding.

Q *Can I breast-feed if I have had previous breast surgery?*

A Most women can. Your plastic surgeon will have avoided cutting your milk ducts during breast implant or reduction surgery. Breast biopsies rarely cause a problem.

Q *Can I breast-feed if my baby was born prematurely?*

A Yes. Some premature infants will not be able to feed right away, though. Have your doctor order you a breast pump in the hospital, so that you can start stimulating your breasts to produce milk. As soon as your baby is ready to eat, you may supply the doctors taking care of him or her with your breastmilk.

Q *I want to breast-feed my baby, but I will have to go back to work in 6 weeks. What can I do?*

A For the first 6 weeks, you can breast-feed your baby all you want. When you return to work, you can use a breast pump to save milk for his or her daytime feedings. Breastmilk can be refrigerated for 24 hours. Storage for longer periods of time can be accomplished by freezing your milk. There will be no loss of nutrients or antibodies when milk is frozen and thawed.

Q *What should I do for cracked nipples?*

A To prevent cracked nipples, wash your breast with water only. Soap can dry out the skin. In New Zealand, mothers pat their breasts dry, express some milk, and let it air dry on the nipples. The fat content in the milk will keep the nipples soft. If your nipples are cracked, apply lanolin or some other commercial breast cream that does not have to be washed off before feedings. If you are allergic to wool, do not use lanolin; it is made from wool.

Q *If I start breast-feeding and decide I want to stop, can I?*

A Yes. You can stop breast-feeding anytime you want.

Q *Which medicines should I avoid when I am breast-feeding?*

A A general rule is that you can take any medicine you were taking while you were pregnant. Very few drugs are contraindicated while breast-feeding. Usually, the amount of drug that passes through the breastmilk is too small to have any effect on your baby. However, before you take any medication, call your pediatrician.

Q *What are the signs of a breast infection?*

A Breast infections or postpartum mastitis may occur at anytime during the months that you breast-feed. You can develop a high fever (101°F to 103°F), and a portion of your breast will become hot, red, and tender.

Q *What is the treatment for postpartum mastitis?*

A This infection is easily treated with antibiotics.

Q *Can I still breast-feed if I have postpartum mastitis?*

A Yes, only one duct is infected. Your baby will not become infected by nursing on that breast.

Q *I want to bottle-feed my baby. What can I use to prevent my milk from coming in?*

A There are two methods for preventing lactation (milk secretion). The first method has been around for hundreds of years and is simple and very inexpensive. Wear a snug-fitting, well-supporting bra (your prepregnancy bra) and *avoid* nipple stimulation. This will prevent lactation, but engorgement (swelling) of your breasts will occur, especially between the 3rd and 5th day after delivery. This engorgement may be very uncomfortable in up to 30% of mothers, but may be controlled with the use of ice packs on your breasts and the use of a mild pain reliever. It will take about 2 weeks for your milk glands to dry up.

The second method involves the use of medicine. There are several different medicines that may be used by your doctor; each medicine has its advantages and disadvantages. The two most commonly used lactation suppression medicines in my area are Deladumone OB and Parlodel. Deladumone OB is administered by an intramuscular injection in the delivery room. Painful breast engorgement may occur in up to 25% of mothers, and rebound milk secretion, 2 weeks later, may occur up to 25% of the time. There are no other side effects. Parlodel is given in pill form and is taken twice daily for 2 weeks, then once daily for an additional week. Painful breast engorgement and rebound milk secretion may occur about 10% of the time. A minority of mothers may experience dizziness and headaches, initially. Nausea may be prevented by taking the Parlodel with meals. Vomiting may occur if alcohol is used on this medication. Parlodel is moderately expensive.

Q *I started breast-feeding, but for various reasons I want to stop. How can I dry up my breasts?*

A There are three possible methods you can use. Wearing a tight, supportive bra, and avoiding nipple stimulation, or Parlodel may be used to suppress lactation once breast-feeding was initiated. The birth control pill may also be used to dry up your milk and as an excellent method of contraception.

Q *If I am bottle-feeding, when will I ovulate and have my first period?*

A Ovulation rarely occurs before 6 weeks after delivery; however, it can occur as early as 3 weeks postpartum. Remember, you do not have to have a menstrual period before your first ovulation.

Q *What is rooming-in?*

A Rooming-in is offered by some hospitals. With this option, you have your baby with you 24 hours a day, and the baby does not go to the nursery. In some hospitals, your baby may be with you only when you are awake. The advantage of the modified plan is that it allows you to rest, take naps, and have visitors during your hospital stay. You will also be able to learn how to care for your baby in the hospital first with the help of the nurses.

Q *Is it common not to sleep the first night after delivery?*

A Yes. Even if you were in labor without sleep the previous night, you may not sleep much the night following delivery. You may be too exalted, too excited, and too happy to sleep. Don't worry, this is very normal. You will sleep well the next night. If it is difficult to sleep the next night—as sleeping in the hospital can be for anyone—ask for a sleeping pill; you will not become addicted, and it will not affect your baby.

Q *What should I do in the hospital?*

A Rest. Labor and delivery can be very strenuous, and you should rest up for your new routine at home. Just stay in bed most of the day with your new baby and continue your bonding, holding and cuddling, and talking to him or her. Nurses will be in and out throughout the day to check your blood pressure, massage your fundus (top of your uterus), note the flow of your lochia, help you with breast-feeding, and answer any questions you may have. Some hospitals have parenting classes or videotapes that you can view.

Q *How long should I stay in the hospital?*

A The length of time spent in the hospital used to be an option for everyone. With the different medical plans now offered, some mothers have to leave the hospital on the first or second day after delivery, even if the baby has to stay a few more days (for example, because of newborn jaundice). Other parents, wishing to conserve their funds, may want to leave the hospital 12 hours after delivery, a plan now offered by many hospitals. Nonetheless, a standard stay in the hospital is 2 to 3 days after delivery. First-time mothers usually opt for the shorter stay, while multiparous (more than one) moms who appreciate the rest would rather stay longer.

Q *Why do I still look pregnant after delivery?*

A The day after delivery your abdomen may still appear to be large, even though the top of your uterus is only up to your navel. Your abdomen may be distended with intestinal gas, which may happen with either a vaginal delivery or a cesarean section. To minimize this, walk around a few times per day, drink prune juice, eat foods high in roughage, and avoid foods that stimulate gas production (broccoli, cabbage, and beans).

Q *Should I have a circumcision performed on my son?*

A Circumcision is a minor surgery performed either by the obstetrician or pediatrician. It involves removing the foreskin from the penis. The procedure is done in the nursery and takes only a few minutes. A circumcised penis is easier to keep clean, because the foreskin does not have to be retracted to be washed. There are some infections that can occur only in uncircumcised penises. Discuss this with your doctor before the procedure. The penis heals quite rapidly in a couple of days. Complications rarely occur.

Q *How do I take care of the umbilical cord?*

A You will notice that the umbilical cord will shrivel up and turn a dark blue or black color. This is normal. After about 7 to 14 days the cord will fall off and be replaced by a belly button. Until the cord falls off, wash it with alcohol every day. This will both dry out the cord and keep it clean. Try not to cover the cord with a diaper, and do not bathe until the cord falls off.

Q *Can I make my baby have an "inny" or "outy" belly button?*

A The type of belly button is predetermined by your baby's genes, just like the shape of his or her nose or color of eyes.

Q *What should I do on the first day I go home?*

A Rest and enjoy your new baby. Many women tire easily from just packing to go home and unpacking when getting home. This is normal. You may not feel up to visitors, so don't invite anyone. If your mother or close relative wants to cook meals for you, great. If you have other children at home, give them a good deal of attention, alone and with their new brother or sister, so they realize that you still love them as much as you did before the new baby came home with you.

Q *How soon after delivery can I have sexual intercourse?*

A If you had an episiotomy, you should wait at least 3 weeks before attempting sexual intercourse. It takes 3 weeks for the incision to heal properly. If you did not have an episiotomy, you may resume sex after 2 weeks. The same goes for after a C/S. Intercourse, however, may be uncomfortable this early, because your vagina has not returned to its former prepregnancy state. The skin in your vagina may be very thin, especially if you are breast-feeding, and not well lubricated. Be careful your first time, use a lubricant, and stop if it is too uncomfortable. Many new parents are too tired to even think about having sex for many weeks after bringing their new baby home.

Most doctors will want to examine you before you resume having sex. Discuss this and contraception with your doctor before you leave the hospital.

Q *What are the postpartum blues?*

A The postpartum blues are a temporary feeling of sadness, fatigue, irritability, sleeplessness, mood changes, and hostility towards anyone and everyone, including your new baby. Postpartum blues are different from postpartum depression, which is a major psychotic illness characterized by confusion, disorientation, hallucinations, loss of all emotions, decreased activity, and a sense of helplessness and hopelessness.

Q *How common are the postpartum blues?*

A At least 80% of postpartum women experience it. It may last only an hour or as long as a week. You may experience the blues anytime from the first day after delivery to 3 months postpartum. Most commonly, this depressed feeling occurs between the 3rd and 5th days postpartum. In contrast, postpartum depression is rare, occurring in 1 of every 1,000 births.

Q *What causes the postpartum blues?*

A No individual factor can be pinned down as the cause. It is a combination of factors:
- The rapid decrease in the levels of the hormones of pregnancy
- The unexpected feeling of fatigue after delivery
- The adjustment to a new sleep schedule, the episiotomy, afterpains, hemorrhoids, constipation, and breast tenderness
- The sense of loss associated with not being pregnant, not being the center of attention, and not feeling "one" with your baby
- The apprehension about the responsibility of being a good mother and not just a milk dispenser.

Q *What should I do if I have the blues?*

A As I mentioned before, the blues are temporary. If you have prepared yourself for them, you will recognize that you are experiencing this feeling and will be more apt to cope with it. Discuss your feelings with your partner, mother, friends, and doctor. They will lend support and reassurance. If you are experiencing insomnia and have not slept for over a day, ask for a sleeping pill and have your partner manage the night feedings. A good night's sleep will leave you refreshed and ready for motherhood.

Q *When can I start exercising postpartum?*

A You may start as soon as you feel up to it. If you were not exercising during your pregnancy, start very slowly, not more than 5 minutes per day, and gradually work your way up to your normal routine. Walking and swimming are excellent methods to slim down your waist. You may start swimming as soon as your bleeding has subsided.

Q *When will I lose the weight I gained during my pregnancy?*

A Following delivery, you will have lost the weight equal to the weight of your baby, placenta, and amniotic fluid. By the end of your first week postpartum, the excess water weight will also be shed. The extra weight of the uterus will be lost by 1 month postpartum. So by your first postpartum visit, without dieting, you will have lost about 80% of the weight you gained during your pregnancy (if you gained the recommended amount of weight).

Q *Are there* warning signs *that I should notify my doctor about during the postpartum period?*

A Yes. If you experience any of the following, call your doctor and don't wait until your postpartum checkup:
- Vaginal bleeding that is a heavy flow of bright-red blood, more than your normal menstrual period
- Increasing tenderness, redness, and warmth in one section of your breast with fever of 100.4°F degrees or above
- Abdominal pain with fever of 100.4°F or above and chills
- Increasing pain and tenderness at the episiotomy site
- Frequency and/or burning with urination
- Dizziness or fainting
- Severe, persistent headache
- Insomnia
- Severe depression

13 Pregnancy in Women over 35

Q *If my partner is 35 or older, does this increase my risk of having a child with Down's syndrome or another congenital anomaly?*

A No. Statistical studies have not shown an independent effect of the father's age on the incidence of congenital defects. Advanced paternal age (over 40) does not increase the incidence of Down's syndrome. The effect of paternal age does increase the risk of new mutations, but by no more than 1%. This is in addition to the 2% to 3% risk of birth defects in any pregnancy.

Q *Is my age a risk factor for having a miscarriage?*

A Yes. Miscarriages in women over the age of 35 are 50% more common than in women between the ages of 20 and 30. Over 40, they are twice as common. However, other factors besides age may be involved.

Q *Does my age increase my risk for having a stillborn?*

A No. The fetus that survives the first trimester is at no greater risk of stillbirth at term, if you are otherwise healthy.

Q *Will my labor be longer if I am 35 or older?*

A No. The length of labor does not seem to be affected by the age of the mother.

Q *Will I have more complications during labor if I am 35 or older?*

A If you are in good health, the course of labor and delivery should be no different than among your younger friends. However, if you are not as physically fit as your younger counterparts or do have medical problems, your chance of requiring a cesarean section for delivery is higher.

Q *What are the medical problems that are more frequent in women over the age of 35?*

A Hypertension, diabetes, heart disease, obesity, and uterine fibroids are all more common in women with advancing age. If you have one of these disorders, consult your doctor.

Q *Is toxemia more common in women over 35?*

A Yes. Toxemia is one and one-half times as common.

Q *Is the risk of having a baby with spina bifida increased if I am 35 or older?*

A No. There does not seem to be an age-related risk.

Q *What is Down's syndrome?*

A Down's syndrome is a chromosomal disorder. Normally each cell has 23 pairs of chromosomes. In Down's syndrome, there is an extra chromosome with the 21st pair. This extra chromosome may cause a variety of abnormalities in the child, such as characteristically distorted facial features (hence, the reason the disorder is named Mongolism), mental retardation, and high incidence of heart abnormalities.

Q *What is the risk of having a baby with Down's syndrome if I am 35 or older?*

A

Frequency of Down's Syndrome

Maternal Age	Infants per Births
30	1/885
31	1/826
32	1/725
33	1/529
34	1/465
35	1/365
36	1/287
37	1/225
38	1/176
39	1/139
40	1/109
41	1/85
42	1/67
43	1/53
44	1/41
45	1/32
46	1/25
47	1/20
48	1/16
49	1/12

Q *How can Down's syndrome be detected?*

A Down's syndrome can be detected by chorionic villus sampling at 9 to 11 weeks or by amniocentesis at 16 to 18 weeks.

Q *Are there many women pregnant over the age of 35?*

A Yes, and the numbers are rising. There are approximately 3 million pregnancies every year, and it has been estimated that the number of pregnancies in women over 35 will be close to 200,000 per year in the United States by 1987.

14 Myths

Q *I heard that when I cough, the baby loses oxygen. Is this true?*

A No.

Q *I heard that if I raise my hands over my head, the umbilical cord will wrap around my baby's neck. Will it?*

A No. The cord wraps around the neck of the fetus because of the sommersaults it does in the first and second trimesters.

Q *Does taking castor oil start labor?*

A No, but you will have a bowel movement.

Q *Does walking for a long time start labor?*

A No, but it is good exercise.

Q *Does a fast heartbeat mean that I will have a girl, or a slow heartbeat mean that I will have a boy?*

A No. The heart rate is the same for male and female fetuses. The heart rate is faster after fetal movement, however.

Q *Does a pregnant uterus that protrudes and is carried low mean that I will have a girl?*

A No. A protruding abdomen occurs if your abdominal muscles are lax.

Q *Will crying or screaming harm my baby?*

A No.

Q *Can my partner's penis hurt our fetus if we make love?*

A No.

Q *What is "dry" labor?*

A There is no such thing.

Q *Does the way the hair grows on the back of my neck reveal the sex of my baby?*

A No. The tale goes as follows: if your hair grows straight, you are having a girl; if the hair grows to a point, you are having a boy.

Q *Will the Drano test reveal the sex of my baby?*

A No. The tale goes as follows: if your urine turns blue with Drano, you are having a girl; if it remains colorless, you are having a boy.

Q *Will the needle-and-thread test reveal the sex of my baby?*

A No. The tale goes as follows: if the needle and thread held over your abdomen turns in a circle, you are having a girl; if it moves up and down, you are having a boy.

Q *Does the fetus take whatever nutrition it needs from me, no matter how I eat?*

A No!

Q *Am I eating for two?*

A No.

Q *If I experience heartburn throughout my pregnancy, will my baby be hairy?*

A No.

Q *Can your uterus get bruised by the fetus kicking?*

A No.

Q *Is it true that the baby is inactive during labor?*

A No. The fetus will move around during labor.

Q *Will eating a lot of sugar during my pregnancy cause my baby to be hyperactive?*

A No, but you and your baby may be overweight.

Q *Will lying on your stomach during pregnancy squash the baby?*

A No.

Index

Abortion, spontaneous, 70–73
Abruptio placenta, 73–74
Acetaminophen, 55
Acid in stomach, 20–21
Acne, 37
ACOG exercise guidelines, 47–48
Active phase of labor, 113
Aerobic exercise, 45
AFP (alphafetoprotein) blood test, 57–58
Afterpains, 139
AIDS (Acquired Immune Deficiency Syndrome), 91–93
Air hunger, 24
Airplane travel, 42
Alcohol, 49–50
Allergies to pets, 41
Alphafetoprotein blood test, 57–58
Amino acids, 33
Amnihook, 128
Amniocentesis, 60–61
    Rh disease and, 82
Amniotic fluid, 9, 60
    premature rupture of
        membranes and, 84

Analgesics for labor, 122–26
Anemia, 19
Anencephaly, 58
Anesthesia
    dental, 39
    episiotomy and, 117
    for labor, 122–26
    spinal, 126
Ankles, swelling of, 26
Antacids, 21
Antigen, Rh, 3, 80
Anxiety
    fetus and, 37
    miscarriage and, 71
Apgar score, 119
Appendicitis, 105
Artificial sweeteners, 35–36
Aspartame, 35–36
Aspirin, 55

Back labor, 128
Back pain, 15–16
Bathing, 37–38
    of newborn, 121
Bed, birthing, 109

159

Belly button, newborn's, 149
Biophysical profile, 60
Birth defects
  medication and, 53
  x-rays and, 56
Birthing bed, 109
Bladder, 13
  infection of, 103
Bleeding
  after sexual intercourse, 44
  painless, 75–76
  postpartum, 139
  See also Complications of
    pregnancy
Blood clots, postpartum, 140
Blood donations, 130
Blood pressure, 18
Blood tests
  alphafetoprotein blood test,
    57–58
  complete blood count, 2
  Rh titer, 3, 82
  for toxoplasmosis, 63
Blood type, 3
Bloody show, 108
Bottle-feeding, 146–47
Bradley method, 5
Bras, 40
BRAT diet, 17
Braxton-Hicks contractions, 14,
  110
Breasts
  bras and, 40
  growth of, 15
  infection of, 145
  pain in, 14
Breast pump, 144
Breast-feeding, 140–47
  AIDS and, 93
  Cesarean section and, 134
  contraception and, 144
  following birth, 120
  stopping, 147
Breathing, shortness in, 24
Breech presentation, 79–80

Caffeine, 52
Caked nipples, 15

Calcium, leg cramps and, 17
Caloric intake, 29
Carbohydrates in diet, 35
Carpal tunnel syndrome, 24
CBC (complete blood count), 2
Castor oil, 155
Cervix
  labor and, 113
  ripe, 108, 129
Cesarean section, 131–37
  breech presentation and, 79
  herpes and, 95
  placenta previa and, 76
  preparations for, 132
  vaginal delivery after, 136
Chair, birthing, 109
Chickenpox, 102–3
Childbirth classes, 5–6
Chlamydial infection, 97–98
Cholasma, 24
Chorioamniotic sac, 9
Chorionic villus sampling (CVS),
  66–68
Cigarettes, 50–51
Circumcision, 148
Classes, childbirth, 5–6
Cocaine, 52
Coffee, 52
Colds, 100
Colostrum, 15
Complete blood count (CBC), 2
Complications of pregnancy, 6
  medical, 91–105
    AIDS, 91–93
    chickenpox, 102–3
    cytomegalovirus (CMV)
      infection, 101–2
    diabetes, 3, 98–99
    herpes, 93–95
    mitral valve prolapse (MVP),
      99–100
    rubella, 102
    urinary tract infections, 103–4
    vaginal infections, 95–98
    viral infections, 100–101
  mother's age and, 153
  obstetrical, 70–90
    abruptio placenta, 73–74

beech presentation, 79–80
ectopic pregnancy, 82–84
intrauterine growth
    retardation, 85–87
miscarriage, 49, 50, 70–73
placenta previa, 74–77
postterm pregnancy, 88–89
premature rupture of
    membranes, 84–85
preterm labor, 87–88
Rh disease, 80–82
toxemia, 77–79
twins, 89–90
surgical, 104–5
Computer terminals, 43
Condyloma acuminata, 97
Constipation, 16–17
Contact lenses, 38
Contraception, breast-feeding and,
    144
Contractions, Braxton-Hicks, 14,
    110
Cooking, microwave, 40
Corneal swelling, 38
Coughing, 155
Cracked nipples, 145
Cramping
  legs, 17
  uterine, 14
Cravings, food, 35
Crowning, 108, 116
Crying, newborn, 119, 156
CVS (chorionic villus sampling),
    66–68
Cyst, ovarian, 105
Cystitis, 103
Cytomegalovirus (CMV) infection,
    101–2

Datril, 55
D&C (dilatation and curettage), 72
Delivery. *See* Labor
Delivery date, 7, 8
Demerol, 123
Dental care, 39
Depression, postpartum, 150
Diabetes, 3, 98–99
Diabetes screening test, 63

Diarrhea, 111
Diet, 28–36. *See also* Nutrition
Dilatation and curettage, 72
Dilation, 107, 113
Dizziness, 18
Douching, 38–39
Down's syndrome, 58
  mother's age and, 152–54
Drano test, 156
Drinking alcohol, 49–50, 71
Drugs, 49–56
  alcohol, 49–50
  illicit, 51–52
  See also Medications

Ectopic pregnancy, 82–84
Edema, 26
Effacement, 107
Electronic fetal monitoring, 64–65
Embryo, development of, 10
Employment, 43–44
Enema, 109
Engagement, 107
Epidural, 124–26
Episiotomy, 116–18
  postpartum care of, 138, 149
Estimated date of confinement, 7,
    8
Exam
  pelvic, 2, 4
  physical, 1
Exercise, 45–48
  ACOG guidelines for, 47–48
  labor and, 46
  level of, 45
  postpartum, 151
External cephalic version, 79
Eyes, newborn's, 120
Eyesight, 38

False labor, 110
Fat in diet, 34
Fatigue, 18–19
Feet, swelling of, 26
Fetal Alcohol Syndrome, 50
Fetal movement test, 68–69
Fetus
  development of, 7–12

heart rate of, 64-66, 156
heart sound of, 4
medicine and, 55-56
movement of, 8, 68-69, 111, 157
noise and, 41
size of, 10-12
stress and, 37
Fever, 101
Fiber in diet, 35
Fingernails, 23
Fingers
  rings and, 40
  tingling in, 23-24
First stage of labor, 112-14
Flatulence, 19
Flu, 101
Fluid consumption, 34
Fluoride supplements, 39
Follow-up office visits, 3
Food groups, 30. *See also*
  Nutrition
Forceps, 115, 126
Fruit in diet, 31-32

Gardnerella vaginalis (G.V.)
  vaginitis, 96
Gas, 19
Genital herpes, 93-95
German measles, 2, 102
Gestation period, 7, 8
Gestational diabetes, 98-99
Gingivitis, 19
Grain in diet, 32
Group B B-streptococcus test,
  61-62
Gums, 19

Hair care, 39-40
Hair growth, 19-20
Hands, numbness in, 23
Headaches, 20
Heart
  exercise and, 48
  fetal, 4, 64-66, 156
  mitral valve prolapse and,
    99-100
  pounding of, 20
Heartburn, 20-21, 157

Hemolysis, 80
Hemorrhoids, 21
Hepatitis B virus screening, 62
Herpes, 93-95
History part of exam, 1
Hospitalization, 111
  Cesarean section and, 135
  packing for, 106
  postpartum, 147
Hot tubs, 40
House pets, 41
Hypertension, pregnancy induced,
  77-79
Hyperventilation, 24

Illicit drugs, 51-52
Immunizations for foreign travel,
  42
Induction of labor, 128-30
Influenza, 101
Insulin, 98-99
Intercourse, 44-45, 156
  after delivery, 149
  AIDS and, 92
Intrauterine growth retardation
  (IUGR), 85-87
Inverted nipples, 140
Iron supplements, 54
Itchiness, 25-26

Jaundice, 80

Kegel exercises, 14
Kidney infection, 104

Labor, 106-30
  active phase of, 113
  back, 128
  classes and, 5
  episiotomy and, 116-18
  exercise and, 46
  false, 110
  fetal monitoring during, 64
  first stage of, 112-14
  hospital procedures for, 111
  induction of, 128-30
  latent phase of, 112
  medications for, 122-26

mother over 35 and, 153
preterm, 87–88
second stage of, 114
signs of, 110
stages of, 112
third stage of, 120
Labor rooms, 112
Lactation, prevention of, 146. *See
also* Breast-feeding
La Leche League, 144
Lamaze method, 5
Latent phase of labor, 112
Leg cramps, 17
Leg pain, 14
Ligaments, stretching of, 14
Linea nigra, 25
LMP (last menstrual period), 7
Local anesthesia, 117
Lochia, 140
Loud noise, fetus and, 41
Lower back pain, 15–16

Marijuana, 51
Mask Of pregnancy, 24
Mastitis, postpartum, 146
Meals
heartburn and, 21
nausea and, 22
See also Nutrition
Measles, German, 2, 102
Meat in diet, 31
Meconium, 127
Medications, 53–56
birth defects and, 53
breast-feeding and, 145
labor and, 122–26
lactation prevention and, 146
over-the-counter, 53
See also Drugs
Megavitamins, 55
Melasma, 24
Membranes, rupture of, 84
Menstrual period
bottle-feeding and, 147
last, 7
Metal detectors, 43
Microwave cooking, 40
Milk in diet, 31

Miscarriage, 70–73
alcohol and, 49
chances of, 73
mother over 35 and, 152
smoking and, 50
Mitral valve prolapse (MVP),
99–100
Morning sickness, 22
Mucous plug, 108
Myths, 155–57

Nagele's rule, 7
Narcotics during labor, 122
Nasal stuffiness, 23
Nausea, 22
Needle-and-thread test, 156
Neural tube defect, 58
Nipple stimulation test, 66
Nipples
changes in, 15
coloring of, 25
cracked, 145
inverted, 140
postpartum care of, 140
sore, 142
Noise, fetus and, 41
Nonstress test, 65–66
Nosebleeds, 23
Numbness in hands, 23
Nurse's role during labor, 119
Nutrition, 28–36
balance in, 33
breast-feeding and, 143
fetal development and, 30, 157
food groups and, 30–33
toxemia and, 78
See also Meals

Office visits, 1–6
follow-up, 3
Oral sex, 45
Ovarian cyst, 105
Over-the-counter medicines, 53
Overweight, 29

Paints, 41
Panadol, 55
Pelvic exam, 2, 4

Permanents, 39
Pesticides, 41
Pets, 41
Phenylketonuria (PKU), 36
Physical exam, 2
Pica, 35
Piles, 21
Pitocin, 108, 130
Placenta, 8, 12
  abruption of, 73–74
  alcohol and, 49
  expulsion of, 120
Placenta previa, 74–77
Plane trips, 42
Postpartum care, 138–51
  bleeding and, 139
  breast-feeding and, 140–47
  depression and, 150
  episiotomy and, 138–39
  exercise and, 151
  hospitalization and, 147
  warning signs and, 151
Postpartum mastitis, 146
Postpartum shakes, 121
Postterm pregnancy, 88–89
Preeclampsia, 77–79
Pregnancy
  complications of. *See*
    Complications of
    pregnancy
  duration of, 7, 8
  ectopic, 82–84
  first, 8
  first month of, 9
  postterm, 88–89
  women over 35 and, 152–54
Pregnancy induced hypertension,
  77–79
Premature infants, 87–88
  breast-feeding and, 144
Premature rupture of membranes,
  84–85
Prenatal office visits, 1–6
Prenatal vitamins, 53–55
Prep, 109
Preterm labor, 87–88
Protein in diet, 33–34
Psychoprophylactic Method, 5

Pudendal nerve block, 117
Pushing during labor, 114
Pyelonephritis, 104

Quantitative Beta HCG test, 72

Recovery room, 121
Rh disease, 80–82
Rh immune globulin, 73, 81
Rh titer, 3, 82
Rings, finger swelling and, 40
Ripe cervix, 108, 129
Rooming-in, 147
Round ligament syndrome, 14
Rubella, 102
  test for, 2

Saccharin, 35–36
Saliva, 26
Salt in diet, 34
Saunas, 40
Screening tests, 4, 62–64
Seat belts, 43
Second stage of labor, 114
Sedatives during labor, 122
Sexual intercourse, 44–45, 156
  after delivery, 149
  AIDS and, 92
Shortness of breath, 24
Show, 108
Skin
  acne, 37
  coloring of, 24–25
  itching of, 25–26
  stretch marks in, 25
Smoking, 50–51, 71
Sodium, 34
Spina bifida, 57, 153
Spinal anesthesia, 126
Spontaneous abortion, 70–73
Sports and exercise, 46
Spotting. *See* Bleeding
Stages of labor, 112
Station, 107
Stillborn, 152
Stress
  fetus and, 37
  miscarriage and, 71

Stretch marks, 25
Sudden Infant Death Syndrome
  (SIDS)
  cocaine and, 52
  smoking and, 51
Sugar, 157
Sunbathing, 38
Surgery, 104-5
Sweeteners, artificial, 35-36
Swelling
  of ankles and feet, 26
Syphilis, 2

Terminals, computer, 43
Tests
  alphafetoprotein blood, 57-58
  amniocentesis, 60-61
  blood, 2, 3, 63, 82
  chorionic villus sampling,
    66-68
  diabetes screening, 63
  electronic fetal monitoring,
    64-65
  fetal movement, 68-69
  group B B-streptococcus, 61-62
  hepatitis B virus screening, 62
  nipple stimulation, 66
  nonstress, 65-66
  quantitative Beta HCG, 72
  rubella, 2
  screening, 4, 62-63
  syphilis, 2
  ultrasound, 59-60
  urine, 3
Threatened abortion, 71
Tiredness, 18-19
Tooth decay, 39
Toxemia, 77-79, 153
Toxoplasmosis, 63-64
Travel, 42
Trichomonal infection, 95
Twins, 89-90
Tylenol, 55

Ultrasound, 59-60
Umbilical cord, 9, 12, 155
  cutting of, 119
  postpartum, 149

Underweight, 29
Urinary tract infections, 103-4
Urination, 13
  bladder infection and, 103
  Kegel exercises and, 14
Urine test, 3
Uterus, measurement of, 4

Vaccines for foreign travel, 42
Vacuum extractor, 115
Vaginal birth after Cesarean
  (VBAC), 136-37
Vaginal bleeding
  after sexual intercourse, 44
  painless, 75-76
  See also Complications of
    pregnancy
Vaginal discharge, 26
Vaginal infections, 95-98
Vaginitis, Gardnerella vaginalis
  (G.V.), 96
Valsalva maneuver, 48
Varicose veins, 27
VDRL, 2
Vegetables in diet, 31-32
Vegetarians, 34
Veins, varicose, 27
Venereal wart infection, 97
Video display terminals, 43
Viral infections, 100-101
Vision, 38
Vitamin A in diet, 32
  fat and, 34
  toxicity by, 55
Vitamin C in diet, 31-32
  iron and, 54
  megadoses of, 55
Vitamin D, 55
Vitamin K, 120
Vitamin supplements, 53-55
Vomiting, 22

Walking, 155
Warning signs, 6
Warts, veneral, 97
Weight gain, 28-30
  distribution of, 29
  See also Nutrition

Weight loss, postpartum, 151
Wharton's jelly, 9
Work, 43–44

X-rays, 56
   dental, 39
Yeast infection, 96